Practical Medical Retina

Practical Medical Retina: Navigating the Net is the third instalment in the 'practical' range to complement *Practical Uveitis* and *Practical Emergency Ophthalmology* books. Medical Retina is one of the largest and most important subspecialties of ophthalmology. Many new and exciting treatments are happening at breakneck speed, making it difficult for ophthalmologists to keep up with developments and understand the best way to treat patients. This book, as with the other two, will provide an easy-to-understand breakdown of developments, a description of current and future therapies, and an accessible assessment of evidence, of which there is currently a bewildering amount.

Key Features:

- Uses algorithms and flowcharts to help with decision-making processes.
- Describes evidence and all relevant papers to understand connections to clinical scenarios for trainees and ophthalmologists.
- Features multiple optical coherence tomography images to better illustrate disease features in an easy-to-understand manner.

Practical Medical Retina
Navigating the Net

Christiana Dinah and Gwyn Samuel Williams

CRC Press
Taylor & Francis Group
Boca Raton London New York

CRC Press is an imprint of the
Taylor & Francis Group, an **informa** business

Designed cover image: Richard Waters

First edition published 2026
by CRC Press
2385 NW Executive Center Drive, Suite 320, Boca Raton FL 33431

and by CRC Press
4 Park Square, Milton Park, Abingdon, Oxon, OX14 4RN

CRC Press is an imprint of Taylor & Francis Group, LLC

© 2026 Christiana Dinah and Gwyn Samuel Williams

ISBN: 978-1-041-04422-2 (hbk)
ISBN: 978-1-041-04420-8 (pbk)
ISBN: 978-1-003-62830-9 (ebk)

DOI: 10.1201/9781003628309

Typeset in Times
by KnowledgeWorks Global Ltd.

Contents

Foreword vii
Acknowledgements ix
Preface xi
Author Biographies xiii

Chapter 1 Introduction 1

Chapter 2 Imaging and Investigations in Medical Retina 3

Chapter 3 Dry Age-Related Macular Degeneration 21

Chapter 4 Neovascular Age-Related Macular Degeneration 36

Chapter 5 Myopic and Other Secondary Neovascular Membranes 62

Chapter 6 Diabetic Retinopathy and Maculopathy 74

Chapter 7 Retinal Vein Occlusions 101

Chapter 8 Central Serous Chorioretinopathy 120

Chapter 9 Inherited Retinal Dystrophies and Genetic Conditions ... 129

Chapter 10 Other Important Medical Retina Conditions 142

Chapter 11 Service Planning 166

Chapter 12 Morality and Ethics in Medical Retina 176

Index 181

Foreword

Professor Bird has helped establish Medical Retina as a recognised ophthalmic speciality we now know and love called Medical Retina. Having worked with eminent ophthalmologists all over the world, he has been working as a professor and consultant at Moorfields Eye Hospital, London, from the 1970s until the present. He has trained numerous generations of Medical Retina specialists, including the authors of this book. He is truly a Titanic figure in the field, having published more than 400 papers and received dozens of awards and honours.

Until relatively recently, ophthalmology was considered a surgical discipline to the exclusion of Medical Ophthalmology as a legitimate sub-speciality designation. From the 1970s, largely due to the influence of Dr. Donald Gass, there has been a gradual but real growth of our specialty of Medical Retina as an approved designation within Ophthalmology. This has been the case in large clinical services in the developed world, but it is less so in countries that possess less mature economies and less well-developed medical services, as well as in areas with sparse populations in the developed world. Lack of access to an up-to-date Medical Retina specialist is further complicated by the rapid expansion of expensive, sophisticated imaging techniques and knowing how to interpret increasingly complex images.

This book has the intention of making the knowledge of this important sub-speciality available to those practitioners without access to Medical Retina expertise who feel the need to expand their knowledge, and to trainees who lack expert teaching in the field. The importance is underlined by the increasing prevalence of diabetes and its ophthalmic complications worldwide, as well as of age-related macular degeneration. The book is written in a manner that is easily comprehensible yet current in its understanding and in interpreting the various imaging techniques. Attention is paid to the principles of the imaging techniques, which helps in image interpretation and understanding of disease. It is hoped that it will also be useful to those in training to get a good grounding in Medical Retina.

Professor Alan Bird

Acknowledgements

Many thanks, indeed, to Christine Kiire, consultant ophthalmologist at Oxford Eye Hospital, England, for her tireless work in proofreading the text of this book and making invaluable recommendations and additions. Her expertise is much appreciated. Thanks also to Mr. Richard Waters, senior specialist ophthalmic photographer at Singleton Hospital, Swansea, who provided the images. Without his pictures, producing this book would have been impossible. Thanks also to Richard Dunn for helping to modify the cover art.

Preface

Medical Retina is the most innovative, exciting and satisfying branch of ophthalmology. We do more good in our speciality than any other per unit time. Every clinic, injection and laser we undertake saves sight, and therefore we, as Med Ret specialists, bear a mantle of responsibility towards humanity that is both rewarding and intimidating at the same time. It is the very fact that what we do carries such worth that makes the prospect of making a mistake so very intimidating.

But fear no more! *Practical Medical Retina: Navigating the Net* has been written precisely to illuminate a rapidly changing landscape and make decision-making easier for trainees and specialists alike. Every important class of condition in our subspeciality is tackled and deconstructed in turn to help readers make good decisions based on logic and common sense. The latest research is described in detail by Christiana Dinah, a top researcher in our field, in an easy-to-read and accessible manner. Here, we cut through the complexity and return to first principles as all good clinical scientists should.

You can dip into this book when you need specific information about a specific condition, or read the whole text from beginning to end for a comprehensive understanding of our craft. We hope that by reading this book, you will be inspired to both understand the current state of knowledge and be tempted to contribute towards the vital research that is constantly being undertaken to improve outcomes for our patients. It is an exciting journey, and we are privileged to be making it with you!

Author Biographies

Dr. Christiana Dinah is the macula service and research lead at Central Middlesex Hospital. She is the Director for Research and Innovation at LNWH and the Director for the newly established NIHR North West London Commercial Research Delivery Centre. She is also an honorary senior clinical lecturer at Imperial College, London.

She completed her Medical Retina fellowship at Moorfields Eye Hospital and then became a consultant at Central Middlesex Hospital, where she set up the award-winning research department.

Dr. Dinah has served as chief investigator or principal investigator in over 25 clinical trials, from Phase I to Phase IV. She has been involved in writing national guidelines, including the NICE guidelines for diabetic retinopathy. Her research interests are in AMD and retinovascular diseases, and she is passionate about patient-centric research design and inclusion in clinical research.

Professor Gwyn Samuel Williams attended medical school at King's College London and completed his ophthalmology training in the Wales circuit. He undertook a year's fellowship in Medical Retina and uveitis at Moorfields Eye Hospital in London, and from June 2016 onwards, he has been a consultant in Swansea, specialising in Medical Retina and inflammatory eye disease. He is an honorary Associate Professor at Swansea University, and from 2020 to 2023, was Llywydd of the RCOphth in Wales and Clinical Lead for Ophthalmology to the Welsh Government. At present, he is Associate Dean and Head of the School of Ophthalmology in Wales. He has a keen interest in reading, writing and hiking through the beautiful Welsh countryside, and was Plaid Cymru's candidate for the 2019 and 2024 elections in his constituency of Swansea West.

1 Introduction

The beginning of the Pixar film *Ratatouille* states that 'the best food in the world is made in France. The best food in France is made in Paris. And the best food in Paris, some say, is made by Chef Auguste Gusteau', Likewise, it can be said that the most interesting and varied branch of medicine is ophthalmology, and the most interesting and varied branch of ophthalmology is Medical Retina. Once upon a time, Medical Retina was a fairly neglected subspecialty of ophthalmology, viewed by some specialists as comparable to ophthalmic ornithology where interesting and varied conditions could be described and categorised, but nothing more; this is now utterly untrue. Since anti-vascular endothelial growth factor (anti-VEGF) agents were launched around 20 years ago, everything has changed. Pharmaceutical companies are now ploughing more money than ever into researching new treatments for conditions that until not long ago had catastrophic outcomes. Neovascular age-related macular degeneration (nAMD), diabetic retinopathy (DR), diabetic macular oedema (DMO) and retinal vein occlusion (RVO) are now treatable conditions with very real prospects of not just preventing further deterioration of vision but actually reversing some of the damage that occurs when eyes are afflicted by these diseases.

It is indeed an exciting time. Whilst the choice of agents was initially limited, we now have a cornucopia of injections to choose from, with aggressive marketing teams vying for our attention at various conferences and meetings. Although in the past a handful of pivotal papers and research works were enough to guide the intrepid Medical Retina specialist through the jungle, we now have important papers released every year, each with a fancy name shortened to some of the most unlikely acronyms possible. It isn't just injections, either. There have been great strides forward in understanding laser therapy, with several new treatment modalities now being utilised to treat common retinal conditions. We have seen great leaps forward in our understanding of inherited eye diseases and what causes the phenotype of these previously unknowable conditions. There is even a gene therapy treatment available now through the National Health Service (NHS) for a specific mutation in the RPE65 gene, and it is hoped and expected that this is just the tip of the iceberg.

There are old foes, such as central serous chorioretinopathy (CSR), that continue to beguile us. There have been many false hopes and blind alleys, but clinicians may have only a sketchy understanding of the truth about the various research studies that have looked into this common but frustrating condition. Other disease entities such as choroidal naevi, tumours and such are also addressed in a more complex manner than before, and what once was simple, perhaps deceptively so, is now more difficult than ever for the non-specialist to understand. Non-invasive imaging system technology has taken off in Medical Retina, providing us with exquisite, microscopic detail at our fingertips. The days of injecting everyone with fluorescein to perform a formal angiogram are consigned to history except for specific cases, at least for now. Perhaps imaging in the future will become so good that, coupled with artificial intelligence, our diagnostic

DOI: 10.1201/9781003628309-1

1

abilities will become more powerful than we ever thought possible. It is an exciting but confusing time, although these two emotions are usually two sides of the same coin.

Public health in ophthalmology has become increasingly important with diabetic retinopathy screening as well as monitoring systems for hydroxychloroquine retinal toxicity (for complex reasons, this cannot be called screening), and now accounts for much time and money in our departments and services. Due to this explosion of work, we found ourselves quite early on at a huge medical manpower disadvantage that no realistic increase in the number of doctors could fill, so we started as a discipline leaning more and more on non-medical practitioners (NMPs). Initially, NMPs were almost all nurses, but they now include optometrists, orthoptists and many other allied healthcare professionals. Seemingly overnight, the Medical Retina consultant was propelled from an old-fashioned one-man (or woman!) band to a General leading a whole army of troops in a suddenly ferocious and ultimately successful battle against blinding diseases that previously had no effective treatment. Service management is now critical in running a medical retina service, and consultants are not traditionally trained in this process, or are perhaps not that good at such tasks.

Clearly, there have been many exponential developments in our field of Medical Retina that have had the dual effect of significantly increasing the excitement of our day job but also causing much bewilderment. Science is becoming increasingly difficult to understand due to its sheer proliferation and the fact that there is so much money involved that various tricks of the trade are used to push messages to us that the data might not robustly support. The very excitement and newness of these developments are at risk of causing so much confusion that ophthalmologists are discouraged from seeking a career in medical retina, rather than being encouraged and enthused. Perhaps the specialty of medical retina, like the Greek Serpent Ouroboros that is depicted as continuously eating its own tail in a cycle of doom, is now also at risk of devouring itself. But fear not! In the same way that Chef Auguste Gusteau produced his handy guide to cooking, *Anyone Can Cook*, so we have produced this book, *Practical Medical Retina: Navigating the Net*.

We aim to demystify and honestly and truthfully describe things as they really are, wading through the swampy deeps and treacherous forests to bring you only what you need to know in this rapidly developing field of Medical Retina. We will describe the important papers and research, which will help you understand the latest evidence base and enable you to hold your own in any conversation with colleagues or drug reps. Anyone can indeed cook, but only the fearless can be great. Whilst we cannot promise to make you fearless, and it could be argued that such a thing would be undesirable in medicine anyhow, we can make you confident in the current state of affairs and through that, all of you will be great. This book is designed to be simply read in a no-nonsense way by the general Medical Retina specialist, and no PhD or research background will be needed to understand things. The 'Christiana Says' sections explain the research in each area in an understandable manner, and we pull no punches in bringing you the unadulterated truth. We will suggest acceptable treatment algorithms and discuss the ethics of the different courses of action. We hope that this book will be useful to you, dear reader, help you understand the current state of play in medical retina, and enable you to successfully navigate past dangerous rocks and shallows. This journey through medical retina is an exciting one, and we are honoured to have you along with us!

2 Imaging and Investigations in Medical Retina

The world of medical retina has changed a lot over the past few years. Gone are the days of fruitlessly straining at an antiquated slit lamp in an attempt to determine whether there is any fluid present at the macula of a patient with cataract who cannot look straight. The stakes were a lot lower in the past, of course because there were precious few treatments for macular oedema available; this is no longer the case. The old Early Treatment of Diabetic Retinopathy Study (ETDRS), regarded by many as Holy Scripture, based examination findings on what could be seen through the ophthalmologist's funduscopy..

There were tests such as fluorescein and indocyanine green angiography (ICGA) of course, colour fundus imaging (non-widefield) and such, but it was the advent of optical coherence tomography (OCT) that really changed the game completely. For the first time, the ophthalmologist had access to an instrument that could see down to the microscopic level, and hedging the bets of semi-guesswork of the past was suddenly over. The balance between art and science in medical retina lurched decisively over to the latter side. The OCT revolution was accompanied by advances in widefield imaging, autofluorescence, OCT angiography (OCT-A), and more. Suddenly, many Medical Retina specialists found themselves far outside their comfort zones due to rapid advancements in technology around them. The resulting rapid advancement in knowledge, in addition to therapeutic advancements, has led to wide-ranging guidelines being updated increasingly frequently, and knowing which tests (including blood tests, blood pressures and glucose measurements) to do and when is an increasing problem. Depending on when books and papers are published, the advice is different. Nobody wants to be left behind! Fear not – we will bring light to the darkness. Before knowing which tests and investigations to order in each eventuality, we must first understand the technology. This is covered in the different chapters.

OPTICAL COHERENCE TOMOGRAPHY

The basic principle of OCT technology need not be understood in detail by the clinician; indeed, it is highly probable that due to the increasing complexity of modern instrumentation only medical physicists truly have a hope of reliably appreciating the principles involved. A small amount of working knowledge is useful; however, it is enough to know that low-coherence light is split into two beams by the aptly named 'beam-splitter'. One beam enters the eye and the other, termed a reference beam, is sent to a mirror. These beams are then reflected, combined in a special detector, and

DOI: 10.1201/9781003628309-2

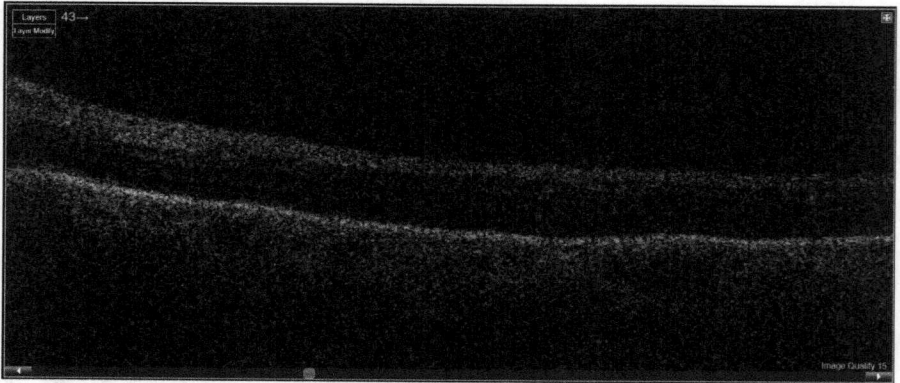

FIGURE 2.1 A time-domain OCT (TD-OCT) image of the retina.

complex maths are utilised to draw an image of the eye by comparing peaks and troughs found in the two signals coming from the two places. The light used is a broad spectrum of frequencies rather than one specific colour alone, which is what 'low coherence' means.

The first generation of OCT machines was called the **time-domain** OCT (TD-OCT). This was because the reference mirror had to move around a bit to capture an image with depth, a process that took time. The pictures were blocky and pixelated by modern standards but at the time represented a miracle of ophthalmic engineering; for the first time in a living patient, layers of cells could be visualised and small amounts of fluid seen and quantified. Figure 2.1 demonstrates the degree of resolution that can be expected from a TD-OCT scan.

The second generation of OCT is called **spectral-domain** OCT (SD-OCT). In this variant, the detector is replaced by a much more powerful device called a spectrometer that can separate the layers without any part of the device having to move. The term 'spectral' is derived from the spectrometer, as opposed to a ghostly apparition, and Fourier (also frequency) was the 19th-century mathematician who invented the actual sums required to determine what the image shows. The images were many times more detailed and powerful than those from TD-OCT; if Medical Retina specialists thought there were no more surprises in store for them in the world of imaging, this leap forward proved them wrong. Figure 2.2 demonstrates the resolution that can be seen in an OCT image.

The third generation of OCT scanning is called **swept-source** OCT (SS-OCT). Very briefly and very simply, instead of simultaneously shining low-coherence light of multiple frequencies, in SS-OCT, a narrow band of light at a specific frequency shines once and then rapidly 'sweeps' through the full frequency range very quickly so that all frequencies are covered but not simultaneously. For very complicated mathematical reasons, this results in a whole different degree of image crispness on a level that takes your breath away. Compared to all previous imaging modalities, SS-OCT is a thing of beautiful detail. Beyond imaging structures that are difficult to see with the human eye in great detail, SS-OCT captures things that have never been

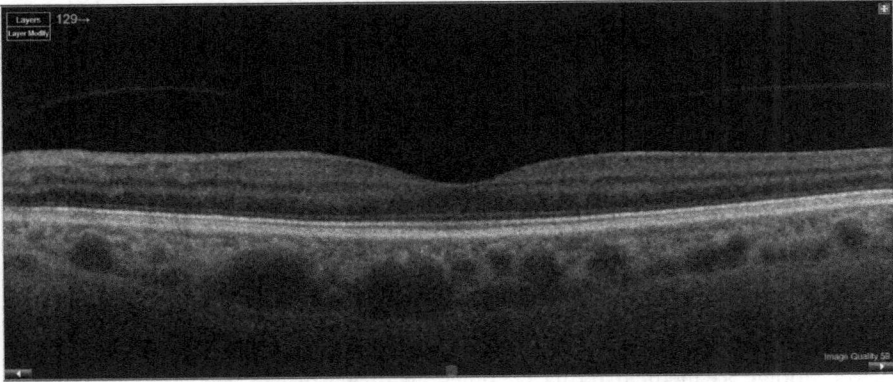

FIGURE 2.2 A Fourier-domain OCT (SD-OCT) image of the retina.

seen by human beings–vitreous opacities, the hyaloid face and deeper structures such as the choroid and posterior sclera. This is demonstrated in Figure 2.3. There are now even more advanced systems with ultrahigh-resolution and higher speeds, that some may call fourth generation.

OCT has changed the face of Medical Retina. It is true that the amount of diagnostic skill required to be a good doctor has now fallen to almost nothing compared to the past. This does not refer to the diagnostic skill required to interpret the clinical picture and formulate a plan. It refers to the skills regarding the tips and tricks for actually seeing the fundus to gain enough raw data for ophthalmologists to know the issues they must address in treatment. One day, the slit lamp will be consigned to a museum alongside other old-fashioned instruments of the quaint old days of medicine. Images from machines are now so much better than those we see ourselves. Moreover, with the development of artificial intelligence algorithms, even interpreting the images and formulating treatment plans are no longer safely in the realm of ophthalmologists, or even human beings more broadly. It is fair to say that this

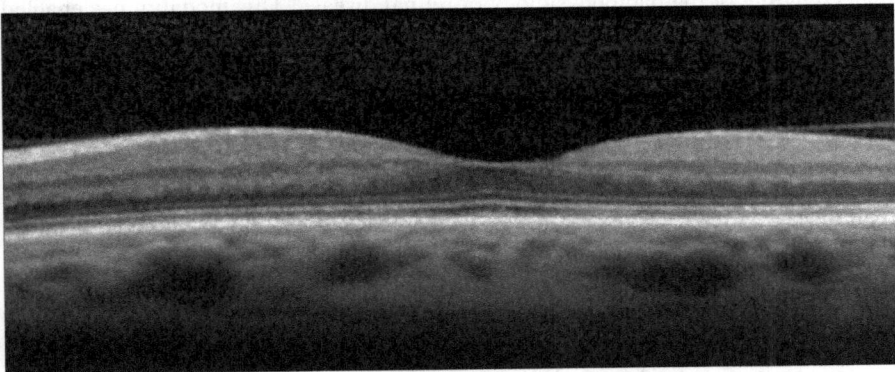

FIGURE 2.3 An SS-OCT image of the retina.

time is not yet upon us, but there are smoke signals on the horizon. It might be that our future role is relegated to simply explaining to the patient what the all-powerful computer has advised in words they can understand like some modern-day Wizard of Oz. However, for now, the slit lamp examination is still part of the theatre of ophthalmology, plays either a political or diplomatic role in the consultation process, or a more practical one if advanced imaging is not yet available.

In the early days of OCT, the cases were chosen carefully because capacity was limited for this new special investigation. However, now it is far more common for every patient in the clinic to be scanned. Of course, this is a double-edged sword because on the one hand, time is not wasted in asking for scans that should have been done initially, but on the other hand, pathologies are found that would have been much better off perhaps undiscovered. There will also be a cost associated with server storage as medical retina becomes an image-driven specialty. The human body is not perfect, and neither is the human eye. Because we were unable to look so deeply into so many eyes until very recently, clinicians around the world are still coming to grips with the appearance of normal variants and various scarring and imperfections. Similarly, patients with conditions such as diabetic macular oedema (DMO) with very good vision are sometimes better off not knowing that they have small clinically insignificant amounts of fluid. 'If you don't take a temperature, you can't find a fever' is a valuable dictum in medicine, and not doing a test can sometimes be the best course if the result does not actually alter what you do. On the other hand, this is indeed a phase we are going through, a learning curve, and once we have enough knowledge of what constitutes normality, we will then be better able than ever before to know the correct course of action. This is particularly the case at present, with OCT scans freely available at many high-street optometry practices for a small additional fee. If the optometrist ordering the test can interpret the result properly, then this is a step forward, but if they cannot, then it is a dangerous step sideways or backwards, resulting in a slew of inappropriate referrals and worry for the patient.

Christiana Says...

OCT provides us with a semi-histological optical biopsy of the macula, allowing intricate detail that not only provides diagnostic insight, but often facilitates an understanding of the pathophysiology of retinal disease. This modality has enabled us to detect precursor lesions for various retinal diseases as well as biomarkers that correlate not only with the presence of disease but also with therapeutic response and prognosis. The non-invasive and rapid nature of OCT acquisition, with an axial resolution as low as 3–5 microns (or even 1 micron in the case of ultrahigh-resolution OCT) has enabled widespread implementation. Importantly, the images obtained improve our ability to classify, predict outcome, facilitate patient understanding of their disease, improving compliance and adherence to treatment plans and follow-up. I will illustrate with some examples below.

OCT Biomarkers in DMO

When examining patients with DMO, many still refer to clinically significant macular oedema, which is a clearly defined diagnostic criteria based on clinical examination alone. With the advent of OCT, many attempts have been made to update the definition of DMO to incorporate OCT because treatment initiation and response assessment is now often based on this technology. Certain OCT features have mounting evidence establishing them as prognostic. These include disorganisation of retinal inner layers (DRIL), disruption of the ellipsoid zone and disruption of the external limiting membrane. Other features are more frequently associated with chronicity, such as outer retinal atrophy, or are more likely to require vitreoretinal surgical intervention, such as vitreoretinal traction or epiretinal membrane. The European School of Advanced Studies in Ophthalmology (ESASO) classification of DMO, for example, is a five-stage OCT-based grading system that may have implications for choice of treatment and treatment response (see Chapter 6). Initial studies using this classification have shown prognostic and therapeutic relevance, but there have been no universally accepted, peer-reviewed validation or utilisation in randomised controlled trials so far (1).

OCT Biomarkers in Proliferative Diabetic Retinopathy

In diabetes, beyond macular oedema, our trusted friend the OCT has utility in detecting proliferative diabetic retinopathy (PDR) by allowing evaluation of retinal neovascularisation at its very earliest stages along with associated vitreoretinal interface changes. With OCT, new vessels at the disc (NVD) appear as coils or tufts of hyperreflective tissue sitting or protruding from the optic disc into the vitreous. These are often not visible on fundoscopy or colour photographs and enable much earlier detection. The earliest stages (subclinical NVD) are seen as looped structures containing small hyporeflective spaces on OCT. These can progress to protrude through the posterior hyaloid and into the vitreous body (2). New vessels elsewhere (NVE) present on OCT as homogenous hyperreflective loops breaching the internal limiting membrane (ILM) and protruding into the vitreous with posterior retinal shadowing (3). The posterior hyaloid serves as a scaffold for NVE development and in most cases is attached or partially detached and tethered to neovascular tissue. Using SD-OCT, NVEs have been proposed to develop in three stages: Stage I consists of the disruption of the ILM, Stage II includes horizontal growth along the ILM, and Stage III comprises multiple breaches of the posterior hyaloid and subsequent linear growth (4).

OCT Biomarkers in AMD

Some characteristic OCT features of dry age-related macular degeneration (AMD) are as follows:

- Drusen: (RPE) elevation with moderate hyperreflectivity.
- Subretinal drusenoid deposits: above the RPE, disrupting the ellipsoid zone and causing undulations.
- Hyperreflective foci are small, well-circumscribed punctate hyperreflective spots in the neurosensory retina. Not associated with blood vessel or exudates, no backshadowing, typically <30 microns. Biomarkers of progression to late-stage AMD from intermediate AMD.

- Nascent geographic atrophy (GA) is a subsidence of the outer plexiform layer and inner nuclear layer; hyporeflective wedge-shaped band in the outer retina, loss or disruption of the ellipsoid zone and interdigitation zone, but the RPE is still intact. A precursor to GA and a marker of risk of progression to GA.

ENHANCED-DEPTH IMAGING OCT

A further adaptation of OCT is enhanced-depth imaging OCT (EDI-OCT). This technique is used to improve visualisation of the choroid. EDI-OCT enables non-invasive, rapid assessment of the choroid using the same equipment with minor adjustment making it very accessible. As we learn more about the role of the choroid in AMD, diabetic retinopathy, and the established role in conditions such as pachychoroid spectrum and uveitis, it becomes an important tool to enable better understanding, diagnosis and management of these conditions. When acquiring EDI-OCT, instead of focusing on the vitreoretinal interface, the OCT device is physically moved closer to the eye. This shifts the zero-delay line deeper into the tissue and results in better signal penetration right into the choroid. Table 2.1 describes the EDI-OCT features of some medical retina conditions.

OCT ANGIOGRAPHY

The natural extension of OCT is into the realms of angiography. Traditional fundus fluorescein angiography (FFA) and ICGA still have a place of course, and will be discussed below, but OCT-A has eaten the heart out of the traditional FFA clinics. The main issue with traditional angiography, apart from the logistical issues and time involved in undertaking the full range of pictures, is the risk. A certain proportion of patients are prone to anaphylaxis, and the risk of death is not zero. OCT-A is a means of visualising the fundal vasculature without that risk. Of course, the downside is that this is **not** a dynamic test measuring fluid leakage but a static test examining architecture. In the case of neovascular AMD (see Chapter 3), OCT-A highlights neovascular membrane complexes but not the state of play with leakage. FFA will demonstrate active leakage if it is present and many other highly important

---

TABLE 2.1

EDI-OCT Features of Some Medical Retina Conditions

Condition	Features on EDI-OCT
Central serous chorioretinopathy (CSCR)	Increased choroidal thickness and dilated Haller's layer vessels
Polypoidal choroidal vasculopathy (PCV)	Choroidal thickening
Vogt–Koyanagi–Harada (VKH) syndrome	Choroidal thickening, reduces with response to treatment
High myopia	Choroidal thinning

signs such as capillary dropout, vasculitis and leakage from new vessels, either at the disc or elsewhere. This is even truer for conditions such as uveitis (see Practical Uveitis for more information).

That said, commonly enough, information is present on the OCT-A to justify commencing the patient on a course of treat-and-extend anti-vascular endothelial growth factor (anti-VEGF) agent and the patient is then spared a potentially risky procedure. OCT-A images are comprised of the OCT itself accompanied by several sections, usually four, at various depths through the retina. Very simply, one looks for the absence of something that should be there or the presence of something that is not. By clicking on each of the four pictures, a coloured slice is displayed over the traditional OCT image indicating the part of the retina to which this picture corresponds, and the borders of this slice can be moved up or down to capture or exclude anything that clinicians wish. This function can be performed to better clarify choroidal neovascular membranes (CNVMs), much like tuning in to various channels with a traditional analogue TV. The one thing that would be even more useful is the ability to draw the segments of the borders ourselves from scratch, but in most cases, this is not possible due to the limitations of both the programming and the technical ability of most ophthalmologists. Figure 2.4 is a normal OCT-A image.

Neovascular complexes can be captured via OCT-A in great detail, though skill is needed to take a good picture. All the toggling of slice borders in the world will do nothing with a bad image, and a clear membrane will remain stubbornly invisible. A skilled operator can also demonstrate the absence of structures such as blood vessels, thereby demonstrating ischaemia without the need for traditional angiography. Diabetic ischaemic maculopathy can be picked up by skilled medical photographers, as well as branch or central vein occlusions. The technology is advancing significantly, and the hope is that as time passes, it can perform an increasing number of the tasks formally requiring FFA or ICG. In each individual chapter on pathologies, the specifics of the OCT-A images will be covered in greater detail.

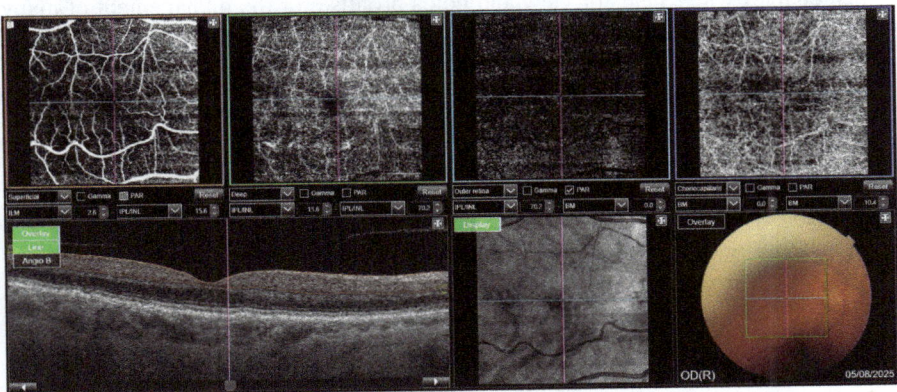

FIGURE 2.4   A normal OCT-A image display.

TABLE 2.2
OCT-A Patterns and Membrane Activity (5)

Pattern	Appearance on OCTA	Activity Status
Medusa/Lacy-wheel	Radiating vessels from the centre	Active, treatment-naive
Seafan	Fan-shaped vessels from one side	Active, often type 1
Ill-defined	Poorly defined, sparse vascular network	Chronic or quiescent CNVM
Dead-tree	Sparse, thick, non-tortuous vessels	Quiescent or post-treatment CNVM

Christiana Says...

OCT-A is built upon the solid immutable foundation of OCT. The advent of OCT and the addition of OCT-A has certainly reduced the use of fluorescein angiography in cases where this was done to confirm the presence of CNVMs before commencing treatment. Whilst OCT-A images require more storage space, may take a little longer than OCT, and can be limited by artefacts from blinking, media opacity or a poor tear-film, these limitations are outweighed by non-invasive, rapid acquisition, which improves patient pathways. CNVM appearances have been classified using OCT-A with wonderfully named patterns denoting active or inactive/post-treatment status. Table 2.2 describes some of these patterns.

OCT-A also allows quantitative analysis of the foveal avascular zone (FAZ) such as area, perimeter and circularity. It has been shown that FAZ enlargement, particularly in the deep plexus, correlates with the severity of diabetic retinopathy, presence and chronicity of DMO and worse visual acuity. There is also emerging evidence that vessel density at baseline may be predictive of treatment response anti-VEGF in DMO (6–8).

Importantly, in many commercial instruments, and in most research studies and clinical practice, OCT-A captures fields of view that are relatively limited compared to fundus photography or fluorescein angiography, for example. Consequently, pathologic features outside this restricted field of view may be missed. In more recent times, some commercial companies have made available ultrawide field OCT-A, which enables wider fields of view and holds promise for the management of many retinal diseases, although this technology is not yet widely available.

WIDEFIELD IMAGING

Most eye departments in the United Kingdom, though not all, now have widefield imaging capabilities. The most common machines in use are Optos systems, though there are others. The technology of the past only enabled the posterior pole or areas reasonably close by to be photographed, but the Optos system allows up to 200 degrees of the retina to be imaged in a single photo. This has many advantages, of course, first and foremost is the ability to capture lesions such as choroidal naevi, tumours and other abnormalities that in the past were too peripheral for a useful photograph to be taken. Monitoring for changes over time or comparing before-and-after images after some intervention is bread and butter for this technology and far exceeds the old system of clinicians having to sketch out on a piece of paper the rough borders

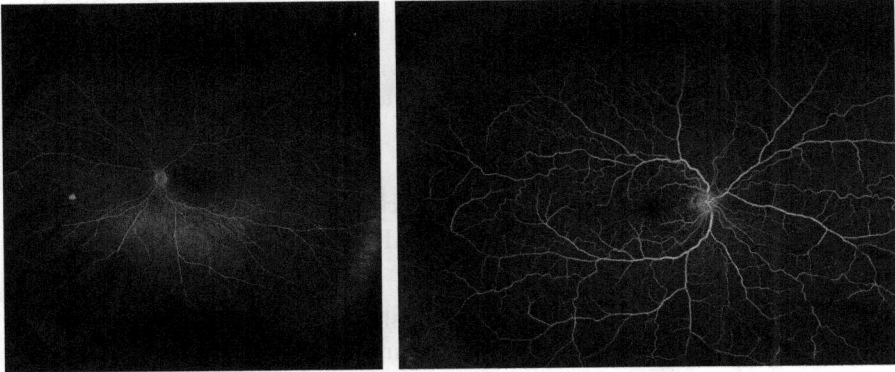

FIGURE 2.5 Widefield fundus fluorescein angiography (FFA).

of a lesion so that another clinician in the future could attempt to deduce whether it had grown or shrunk in size.

Combined with traditional angiography, widefield imaging is much more powerful. Planning targeted panretinal photocoagulation (PRP) in diabetic retinopathy (DR) or retinal vein occlusion can be done with ease using widefield technology. Diagnostic conundrums can also be solved that in the past required pictures to be taken while asking the patient to look in a difficult direction, resulting in one-half of a decent image for every eight blurry ones. In the field of uveitis, FFA and ICG combined with widefield imaging can make all the difference in diagnosing conditions and mapping severity or progression. The images themselves are also very beautiful. Figure 2.5 displays an image of an FFA run in a normal patient. The eyelashes can sometimes be a bit of an annoying issue.

Christiana Says...

Much of what we understand about the clinical features of DR and the natural history of the disease is from clinical observations and standard field fundus photography. The seven fields of the ETDRS standard cover approximately 75–80 degrees of the retina. Widefield fundus photography covers approximately 200 degrees of the retina, providing visualization of the peripheral retina. This has clinical significance in DR because we now know that a proportion of proliferative lesions occur outside the standard seven fields. Protocol AA, a 4-year prospective, multicentre, observational study conducted by the Diabetic Retinopathy Clinical Research Network (DRCR.net) evaluated whether lesions predominantly in the periphery on ultra-widefield (UWF) imaging enhanced prediction of disease progression beyond traditional Diabetic Retinopathy Severity Score (DRSS) grading using seven-field imaging. The study found that UWF fundus imaging revealed more peripheral lesions and led to higher DR grading in 10–12% of eyes, though it did not correlate with increased progression risk. However, peripheral lesions identified on ultra-widefield fluorescein angiography (UWF-FFA) did correlate significantly with progression or need for treatment (9, 10). These eyes, with predominantly peripheral lesions, had a 1.7- to 1.99-fold higher risk of DR worsening over 4 years, independent of other factors. UWF-FFA has also enabled us to rethink how we classify at-risk eyes with central retinal vein occlusion (CRVO) and branch retinal vein occlusion (BRVO), which we delve into the retinal vein occlusion (RVO) chapter. These findings have led to clinical guidance recommending the use of widefield imaging for diagnostic and monitoring purposes (National Institute for Health and Care Excellence [NICE] guidance) (11).

FUNDUS FLUORESCEIN ANGIOGRAPHY
AND INDOCYANINE GREEN ANGIOGRAPHY

Whilst this diagnostic tool is not new and can be used for multiple medical retina conditions, it is indeed true that its territory is shrinking. One day, OCT technology may well reduce this to nothing or almost nothing; indeed, there is a question tabled at many retinal meetings on whether the days of true angiography are numbered. It has been striking how, in the bread-and-butter FFA territory of neovascular AMD, there has been an almost total collapse in angiograms performed in favour of OCT-A, though for now, there is still a viable habitat for this medical retina dinosaur.

Christiana Says. . .

As previously stated, UWF-FFA can predict a higher risk of progression in some patients with diabetes. This is largely related to this modality's ability to detect larger areas of capillary non-perfusion. The same principle applies in sickle cell retinopathy, RVO and other ischaemic retinovascular diseases. As UWF-OCTA technology improves, it may be able to detect capillary non-perfusion comparable to traditional FFA and has the added advantages of visualizing the deep capillary plexus, being non-invasive and requiring less skill and staffing resources. In addition, there are early prototypes that visualise leakage using modified OCT technology. Until then, FFA remains an important diagnostic modality. ICGA is less frequently used, though this may contribute to the under-diagnosis of conditions such as idiopathic polypoidal choroidal vasculopathy (IPCV), where the flow within polyps can be too slow to be detected by OCT-A. I do agree that the speed of advancement in retinal imaging suggests dye angiography as we know it may soon become obsolete.

FUNDUS AUTOFLUORESCENCE

Fundus autofluorescence (FAF) imaging is essentially a picture of the health of the RPE; an RPE-o-gram. It does this by measuring naturally occurring fluorophores in the eye, mainly lipofuscin, that live in the RPE. The optic disc has no RPE and is therefore black on FAF imaging, as are blood vessels, because they block the glow from the underlying RPE. Black areas indicate areas of RPE atrophy or some sort of masking defect due to various sorts of haemorrhages, for example, and can be used to measure progression of conditions such as GA.

Hyperautofluorescence, by contrast, can indicate RPE working overtime, and this usually occurs at the edges of areas where the RPE cells have died as photoreceptors, and desperate to stay alive, try to plug into adjoining RPE cells to recycle the waste. Abnormal fluorophores, such as vitelliform lesions or optic nerve head drusen, also glow brightly on FAF. The main advantage of this test over true angiography is the fact that dye injection is not needed; therefore, avoiding all the potential issues and

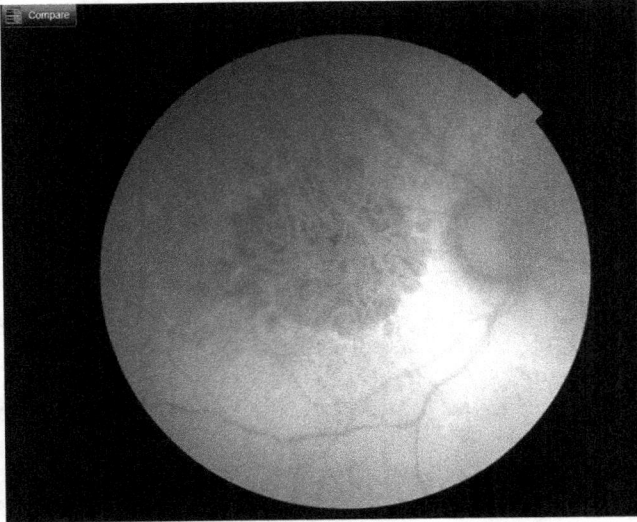

FIGURE 2.6 Fundus autofluorescence (FAF) of a patient with atrophic, or dry, age-related macular degeneration (AMD).

problems with anaphylaxis and other side effects. It is particularly good for seeing what the human eye and regular colour fundus imaging cannot, and in assessing patients with underlying genetic or chronic conditions such as CSCR. In simple terms, black areas on FAF indicate 'dead' and bright areas indicate 'dying'.

Figure 2.6 displays the FAF of a patient with dry macular degeneration. This would have been the main use for this technology by far had the GA injection treatment with various complement inhibitors been licensed for use in the United Kingdom and Europe, but for better or worse, this was not to be.

Christiana Says...

This simple test can provide very useful insights for Medical Retina specialists going through the investigative process of determining the underlying cause of their patient's complaint. There are different types of FAF, with subtle differences that can result in the image being more or less informative depending on the disease being evaluated. The differences are due to the excitation wavelength used. Most common is short wavelength autofluorescence (excitation at 488-nm blue light). The fluorophore (the molecule that absorbs light at a specific wavelength and then emits light at a longer wavelength) is lipofuscin in the RPE and is ideal for use in AMD, inherited dystrophies and so on. With green wavelength autofluorescence (excitation at 504- to 532-nm green light), the fluorophore is also lipofuscin in the RPE though with less absorption by macular pigments, making it more helpful when assessing the foveal region. Finally, near-infrared autofluorescence, with an excitation of 787 nm and fluorophores of melanin and melanolipofuscin in the RPE and choroid, highlights melanin-rich tissues and may be useful in earlier detection of GA and inherited retinal dystrophies (12). It is a simple though wondrous test!

ELECTROPHYSIOLOGY

Measuring retinal electricity is a way of exposing underlying dysfunction of specific cells, rods or cones and assessing the function of the macula, optic nerve and retina as a whole. Electroretinograms (ERGs) measure the potentials generated by the retina as a whole, with multifocal ERGs being useful in demonstrating specific areas of dysfunction. Cone flicker isolates the action of cones, as you'd expect, and visual evoked potentials (VEPs) combined with pattern ERGs can assess the functionality of the optic nerve. The electrooculogram (EOG) measures the standing potential of the eye as a whole and is stated as a ratio, the Arden Ratio of the light peak to the dark trough with a normal result being greater than 1.8. This test is useful in measuring a whole host of genetic conditions that can affect the eye, as well as poisonings and uveitic conditions. A phenomenon called electronegativity also occurs in an ERG when there is inner retinal dysfunction, again, caused by a list of conditions that are only really remembered for exam purposes.

In reality, electrophysiology is ordered by ophthalmologists when we suspect genetic causes for visual dysfunction, to monitor certain inflammatory conditions such as birdshot chorioretinopathy or if we don't know what's going on, can't see a problem, and want to rule out any underlying condition. Again, in reality, the complex waves produced by these tests cannot be understood with any accuracy by the common or garden-variety Medical Retina specialist, but many centres still humour us by sending us the full report replete with all the printouts. Many of us then spend what we consider a respectable amount of time looking at these traces while pretending to understand their significance, and then simply skip to the end to read the report. The two or three sentences at the end of a sometimes many-page report are by far the most important here. We do, of course, need to distinguish as well between retinal causes of visual loss and neurological ones.

Electrophysiology tests are difficult to do well, and therefore labs with rigorous standards must be employed to carry them out; this can mean referring the patient to a centre of excellence quite far away. The tests take hours to perform and involve probes and electrodes stuck over various parts of the head and on the cornea itself. This is a precious resource, is onerous for the patient and the electrophysiologist to perform, and shouldn't be undertaken lightly.

VISUAL FIELD TESTS

You might be forgiven for thinking that visual field testing is not in the realm of medical retina and is more the purview of the glaucoma specialist. It must also be remembered, however, that medical retina patients can and do also have issues with pressure control; particularly uveitis patients. Patients with inherited retinal dystrophies such as retinitis pigments can be monitored and followed up with field testing; this does not alter the final outcome of course but will enable some sort of prognostic prediction to be made and to ascertain if driving standards are being met. In the context of white dot syndromes, a visual field test can reveal an enlarged blind spot or larger affected area in conditions such as acute zonal occult outer retinopathy (AZOOR). This might not be a common test for us, but it is still a very useful one.

One scenario where Medical Retina specialists will usually discuss visual field tests is when undertaking PRP for diabetic retinopathy. PRP may negatively impact the visual field and in some cases lead to loss of enough field to drive. The incidence of driving visual field loss is less with the advent of multispot laser for PRP. This is because the traditional argon short wavelength laser with longer duration results in more thermal diffusion and collateral damage and expansion of laser spot size over time, almost like some sort of smart missile barrage relative to carpet bombing from 30,000 feet. Diabetic patients must inform the Driver and Vehicle Licensing Agency (DVLA) when they have had PRP in both eyes or PRP in their only functioning eye.

BLOOD TESTS

Less is more here. Blood tests are useful for a whole host of reasons and are required in many conditions. The Royal College of Ophthalmologists (RCOphth) advises certain blood tests for retinal vein occlusions, for example; a full blood count (FBC), erythrocyte sedimentation rate (ESR) and glucose, as well as a blood pressure test. Perhaps these guidelines will be updated in the future to include a lipid profile. Specific tests will be discussed in detail in the various chapters associated with specific conditions. It is highly tempting, while ordering these tests, to tick every box because the patient 'is having a blood test anyway, so might as well'. No! This is wrong. Blood tests can just as easily deceive as they can help. Any test is considered normal if it falls within a range of normality determined by 95% of the population; for example, the p value is >0.05. Therefore, if 20 different tests are undertaken, it might be expected by chance that one is in the abnormal range, and if a hundred different blood tests are taken, there is a near certainty that several will be highlighted in glaring red. While this can simply be inconvenient most of the time, if a wrongly ticked thyroid function test turns out abnormal, you have to spend time sorting out that issue, even though it had nothing to do with the reason the patient came to see you in the first place. Sometimes they can cause real harm by leading you down a garden path.

Tests that have low sensitivity or specificity are especially bad. Double-stranded DNA or autoantibodies are notorious for misleading ophthalmologists, and there must be a whole host of angry rheumatologists spread liberally across the world who question, with anger, why such a non-specific test was ordered in the first place. This must be especially galling because the eye specialist, having failed to understand the context of the positive test, dumps the problem on an innocent doctor in another specialty. This is exactly why guidance occurs; to avoid pain and suffering for both patients and doctors. Order only what changes management. With blood tests, it is especially easy for us to get dangerously out of our depth as we recklessly tick every box with wild abandon. Remember also that the clinician who orders the test is responsible for what is revealed as well. It is a medicolegal nightmare.

BLOOD GLUCOSE

A pinprick glucose test, commonly called a 'BM' test, does not, in fact, stand for 'blood monitoring' of glucose but the company that made the strips a few decades ago, Boehringer Mannheim. This has a place in diabetic eye clinics where the blood glucose is suspected of being high and is useful in encouraging our diabetology colleagues to get an unstable situation back under control. If a patient with diabetes is behaving peculiarly in clinic, this simple test can also mean the difference between life and death.

BLOOD PRESSURE

Measuring blood pressure is essential in certain conditions and in certain circumstances. Vein occlusion patients, for example, always need their blood pressure measured, and it is one of those rare times when ophthalmologists can pick up a life-threatening situation. One of the authors remembers well how a patient attending the eye casualty department with a branch vein occlusion had been referred, to the medical retina clinic. However, by the time they arrived there a few weeks later, they had suffered a haemorrhagic cerebrovascular accident caused by malignant hypertension. The blood pressure had not been taken in the eye casualty department. Likewise, starting certain medications that are known to affect blood pressure would need a baseline blood pressure to be taken and monitoring at certain stages as well. Guidelines exist for a reason.

That said, the process of measuring blood pressure is cumbersome and if it were undertaken in each and every patient regardless of need, you'd soon run into problems due to false positive results causing work and spreading anxiety. Do *only* what you need to do, but always do what you need to do. As a general rule, any blood pressure of less than 200/100 can be dealt with by referral to the GP and encouraging the patient to follow up your letter within 2 weeks. Sometimes it is useful to write the blood pressure on a piece of paper to give the patient, and it can be surprising what numbers patients can recall. If the blood pressure is higher than this, either systolic or diastolic, then a referral right away to the medical team is the best course of action. Whilst ophthalmologists are indeed doctors, we would not recommend interfering in a domain outside our area of expertise. We would then become responsible for follow-up and monitoring the blood pressure as well, with all the associated issues that failure to do so would involve.

URINE DIPSTICK

This is a rare thing to do in an eye clinic. The most common cause for asking for this test is if a diabetic patient's glucose is suspected of being out of control, but a quick blood glucose test via pinprick is better here. A patient with suspected endogenous endophthalmitis might benefit from a urine dipstick if an infection is suspected as the cause of sepsis, but should the result be positive, care should be swiftly handed over to those medics who know what they're doing with this sort of thing. Uveitis specialists might consider this test in associated conditions that can affect the kidneys, but again, the circumstances should be rare. Eye clinic nurses usually select a career as an ophthalmic nurse to avoid contact with nasty bodily fluids, and if you were to order this test regularly, it would only be a matter of time before you'd instigate a riot. The urine dipstick can also be used to check for pregnancy, which might be an issue in young women of childbearing age, perhaps needing to start an anti-VEGF agent. That said, an eye clinic finding out a patient is pregnant must surely be a very rare event indeed.

Christiana Says...

Ophthalmology clinics often exist in silos, almost as though the eye is an organ that functions independent of the rest of the body. Certainly in medical retina, many of the diseases we manage have systemic aetiologies or contributory factors, and access to insights on systemic parameters supports holistic management of the patient. For example, fenofibrate has recently been demonstrated to reduce the risk of progression of DR (13). A cheaply available treatment, the potential impact on reducing the number of referrals from DR screening programs can be consequential. There are cautions, however, because dose adjustment is required in patients with renal impairment, it is contraindicated in those with liver dysfunction, and renal profile and liver function tests (LFTs) need to be checked every 3 months in the first 12 months of treatment and periodically thereafter and if the patient reports any symptoms.

Another common ailment, hypertension, has an additive deleterious effect on endothelial dysfunction in the context of diabetes, and it is therefore important to counsel our diabetic patients accordingly. Preventing development and progression of DR involves not just glycemic control, but blood pressure and dyslipidemia can also contribute to progression (14, 15). Renal failure can also contribute to macular oedema, which may resolve when fluid overload is addressed.

Furthermore, there is now a pipeline of oral or systemically delivered treatments for retinal diseases that will require holistic management at initiation and for ongoing monitoring. Clearly, medical retina services need to have access to primary care (and relevant secondary care) records to make sure the treating ophthalmologist is aware of contributory systemic conditions and management is seamless, and vice versa. Synchronised electronic medical records could facilitate this and avoid fractures in care that may occur when medical retina services are isolated from general medical care.

B-SCAN ULTRASOUND

The 'B' in B-scan ultrasound actually stands for 'brightness'. The brightness is related to the reflectivity of tissues sending signals back to the probe. This differentiates it from the 'A' scan, which stands for 'amplitude' and is of course a two-dimensional scan with peaks of various amplitudes along the y-axis depending on their relative reflectivity. B-scan ultrasound is usually undertaken by Medical Retina specialists in the context of vitreous haemorrhages or dense vitritis or indeed anything that fills up the eye and prevents proper view of the retina and posterior pole. A diabetic patient with a vitreous haemorrhage, for example, would need a B-scan to make sure the retina hasn't come off. This needs to be clearly documented in the notes. There are many other uses for ultrasound of course; dense cataracts, possible optic nerve head drusen and melanomas. These will be covered in the relevant chapters.

B-scan ultrasound is undertaken by using a probe marked with a line indicating the structures displayed on the upper aspect of the screen. A foot pedal is used to freeze images so they can then be printed or thicknesses measured. In the context of scleritis, B-scanning is used to look for fluid in the sub-Tenon space, referred to as a 'T-sign', due to the interaction of the black line of fluid intersecting the optic nerve.

COMPUTERISED TOMOGRAPHY (CT) AND MAGNETIC RESONANCE IMAGING (MRI) SCANNING

Formal imaging studies such as computerised tomography (CT) and magnetic resonance imaging (MRI) have a role in medical retina in the context of looking for intracranial pathologies that might be correlated with intraocular diseases. This might include lymphoma, demyelinating disease, caroticocavernous fistula, various other vascular disorders, and potential inherited conditions of the ocular tissues. An MRI is usually much more useful than a CT scan, although the wait is longer and as such, CT scanning is usually undertaken in the context of an acute presentation if rapid acquisition of information is needed. Likewise, the use of contrast makes the images far more powerful, though again, limits the speed at which they can be undertaken.

LUMBAR PUNCTURE

This is certainly not a test undertaken by ophthalmologists, but it is important to understand when to ask our medical registrar colleagues to undertake it. By far, the most common ophthalmic reason might well be secondary to swollen discs, which might be due to increased intracranial pressure, with many other medical retina conditions also presenting with potential swollen discs; RVOs or diabetes, for example. There is an overlap of sorts between medical retina and neuro-ophthalmology, so a working knowledge of lumbar puncture is useful.

In some cases of infectious or inflammatory retinitis, neuroimaging and lumbar puncture may be indicated to detect central nervous system (CNS) involvement. These can include life-threatening scenarios, such as where there are atypical retinal infiltrates and there is suspicion of CNS lymphoma. The work-up in these cases is extensive but may include MRI of the brain, which may show periventricular or deep white matter lesions and a lumbar puncture for **cerebrospinal fluid (CSF) cytology** and **flow cytometry** to detect lymphoma cells.

VITREOUS AND AQUEOUS TAP

Used mainly for uveitic conditions, including infective endophthalmitis, it is important to know how to perform both a vitreous and aqueous tap to safely obtain samples of intraocular fluids for testing. More details on these important investigations can be found in *Practical Uveitis*.

Christiana Says...

This is a very important investigative procedure for the Medical Retina specialist. All injection services must be able to promptly perform a vitreous tap and injection of antibiotics in cases of suspected infectious endophthalmitis. Whilst the yield is moderate in most cases (40–70%), acquiring an adequate volume helps to increase this; it is therefore important to be confident in performing this procedure. The rates of endophthalmitis reported after intravitreal injection are very low, approximately 1 in 3500 in most services. However, prompt treatment can prevent devastating consequences. It is also important to recognise that the general population risk of endophthalmitis may be low, but there are some patient populations that may have a higher risk profile such as dementia patients who may not cooperate with post-injection instructions or report symptoms early, or patients with poor lid hygiene or who reside in institutional settings.

Of the pantheon of imaging and investigations available at our disposal in the world of medical retina, the OCT scan is our closest friend and most stalwart ally. It is what defines us as a subspecialty. Of course, all the other tests have their place and all are important in their proper context, but no other test is as commonly or relentlessly performed in our service than the OCT scan. Indeed, we forget how good we actually are at understanding and appreciating this simple test, as when we get referrals from senior colleagues in other subspecialties questioning the presence or absence of neovascular AMD, for example. Sometimes we marvel at why others would come to such wild and fanciful conclusions when the evidence there on the scan is so apparently plain and simple to see. We are lucky to live in this modern world of imaging and investigations but also have to be cautious about using these powerful tools judiciously. A false positive can cause a world of pain to both patient and ophthalmologist. We will now look at the important conditions of our specialty in turn, in which these very important tests all play a vital part.

REFERENCES

1. Panozzo G et al. An optical coherence tomography-based grading of diabetic maculopathy proposed by an international expert panel: The European School for Advanced studies in ophthalmology classification Eur J Ophthalmol. 2020; 30(1):8–18.
2. Muqit MM et al. Fourier-domain optical coherence tomography evaluation of retinal and optic nerve head neovascularisation in proliferative diabetic retinopathy. Br J Ophthalmol. 2014; 98:65–72.
3. Pan J et al. Characteristics of neovascularisation in early stages of proliferative diabetic retinopathy by optical coherence tomography angiography. Am J Ophthalmol. 2018; 192:146–156.
4. Lee CS, Lee AY, Sim DA et al. Reevaluating the definition of intraretinal microvascular abnormalities and neovascularization elsewhere in diabetic retinopathy using optical coherence tomography and fluorescein angiography. Am J Ophthalmol. 2015; 159:101–110.e1.
5. Coscas GJ et al. Optical coherence tomography angiography versus traditional multimodal imaging in assessing the activity of exudative age-related macular degeneration: a new diagnostic challenge. Retina. 2015; 35(11):2219–2228.
6. Elnahry AG. Optical coherence tomography angiography biomarkers predict anatomical response to bevacizumab in diabetic macular edema. Diabetes Metab Syndr Obes. 2022 Feb 9; 15:395–405.
7. Chouhan S et al. Preliminary report on optical coherence tomography angiography biomarkers in non-responders and responders to intravitreal anti-VEGF injection for diabetic macular oedema. Diagnostics. 2023; 13(10):1735.

8. Massengill T et al. Response of diabetic macular oedema to anti-VEGF medications correlates with improvement in macular vessel architecture measured with OCT angiography. Ophthalmol Sci. 2024: 4(4):100478.

9. Silva PS et al. Association of ultra-widefield fluorescein angiography identified retinal nonperfusion and the risk of diabetic retinopathy worsening over time. JAMA Ophthalmol. 2022; 140(10):936–945.

10. Silva PS et al. Diabetic retinopathy lesion types and distribution on ultrawide field imaging and the risk of disease worsening over time. Retina. 2025; 45(1):44–51.

11. National Institute for Health and Care Excellence (NICE). Diabetic Retinopathy guidelines. NG242. 2024. Available at: Overview | Diabetic retinopathy: management and monitoring | Guidance | NICE

12. Kellner S et al. Near-infrared autofluorescence: early detection of retinal pigment epithelial alterations in inherited retinal dystrophies. J Clin Med. 2024; 13(22):6886.

13. Preiss D et al. Effect of fenofibrate on progression of diabetic retinopathy. NEJM Evid. 2024; 3(8):EVIDoad2400179.

14. UK Prospective Diabetes Study Group. Tight blood pressure control and risk of macrovascular and microvascular complications in type 2 diabetes: UKPDS 38. BMJ. 1998; 317(7160):703–713.

15. Wong TY et al. Three-year incidence and cummulative prevalence of retinopathy: The atherosclerosis risk in communities study. Am J Ophthalmol. 2007; 143(6):970–976.

3 Dry Age-Related Macular Degeneration

For a long time, there was nothing much that could be done about non-neovascular, or dry, macular degeneration, and so it was largely neglected by Medical Retina specialists specifically, and ophthalmologists, generally. There were, of course, some hocus-pocus theories over the years concerning lasers and such, and the famous age-related eye disease (AREDS) studies demonstrated a moderate effect in a sub-group of people. This launched a multi-million-pound vitamin industry aimed at, and used by, consumers who would have been outside the subgroup benefitting the most anyway, but until recently, there was nothing concrete that could be done. Now there is, in the form of complement inhibitors. However, there turned out to be a significant catch with these inhibitors and for multiple reasons, they are not licensed in Europe, the United Kingdom, and other places, and are only available in specific locations worldwide. So what's the clear, unvarnished truth about so-called dry macular degeneration? Before we can understand what can be done, we must first understand what it is.

WHAT IS 'DRY' AGE-RELATED MACULAR DEGENERATION?

Dry age-related macular degeneration (AMD) is as inevitable as death or taxes. The only way of avoiding it is by dying young, but if anyone lives to be old enough, the spectre of dry AMD will, in the end, inevitably manifest itself. At least for most of us mere mortals. It is, put simply, the inevitable ageing change of the human macula. The word 'dry' means that it is not leaking fluid, not leaking blood. For this reason, it is also called 'non-exudative' or 'non-neovascular', but it is true that the term 'dry' does lead to a whole host of problems with patients who confuse this with dry eye, which is also sort of inevitable with age as well. It is true that AMD does indeed affect certain families more than others, including most of the entire European race if you consider that a form of extended family, and that some form of genetics is responsible for this. Clinical features involve the presence of drusen, pigment change at the macula, areas of atrophy or any combination of these three.

So what's drusen? It is derived from the German word for 'geode', those crystals that occur inside rocks that form the common staple of museum gift shops world-wide. Drusen was named by Heinrich Müller, who could see them, but did not, and could not, understand their nature; he did, indeed, observe that they 'glittered' as geodes do. Much can be said about the actual histology of drusen other than know-ing that they are simply accumulations of retinal waste products between Bruch's membrane and the retinal pigment epithelium (RPE), which would be irrelevant to

DOI: 10.1201/9781003628309-3

the simple clinician. As the retina ages, it can process waste less effectively and so sweeps dust under the rug rather than carrying it out of the parlour in a dustpan, and eventually the rug becomes lumpy. These lumps are drusen. If they are smaller than the width of an artery as it crosses the disc margin (63 microns), they are called 'small' drusen, and if they are between 63 microns and the size of a vein as it crosses the disc margin (125 microns), they are termed 'intermediate' drusen. Any drusen larger than this are called, as by now should be expected, 'large' drusen. Most often, they are greyish-white clumps and in fact, despite the name, only rarely glisten like geodes. As the drusen grow larger and start to coalesce, the chances of subsequent collapse into geographic atrophy (GA) or secondary choroidal neovascular membrane formation increases. Figure 3.1 depicts typical drusen.

What about pigment change at the macula? If the RPE is lifted off by drusen, then it can start to disintegrate. The pigment, which accounts for the 'P' in RPE, starts to clump together as dots of blackish material at the macula, which can sometimes be confused with blood. Indeed, it is not uncommon to get referrals from optometrists claiming blood at the macula, when the confused ophthalmologist sees only clumps of pigment. It is a sign of RPE sickness that this clumping occurs. That sickness is in part tied to any drusen that cluster below that layer, slowly but surely strangling the oxygen and nutrient supply getting through from the choroid. Sometimes so much dust can accumulate under the rug that the rug itself starts falling apart. This can result in an ischaemic drive in which vascular endothelial growth factor (VEGF) is released by starved cells and blood vessels come to the rescue; this is neovascular AMD and is covered in the next chapter.

What can happen instead is a collapse of the dying cells and conversion into patchy areas of atrophy that slowly grow over time. This is termed GA of the various well-defined patches of RPE, and therefore the overlying photoreceptor death looks like the edges of continents viewed from space. This is a form of advanced AMD and is a process driven by complex biochemical reactions that are in part mediated by genetics and in part by a form of inflammation in which the complement system plays a part. It is for this reason that exploration into the world of complement inhibitors resulted in the development of some treatment modalities. Figure 3.2 demonstrates the growth of GA in an eye over time.

All this was known before the miracle that is optical coherence tomography (OCT) came along, and because Medical Retina specialists always enjoy introducing new terminology from time to time (if you can't fix it, you might as well redefine the problem), there now exist new buzzwords that you should know. Outer retinal atrophy on OCT scanning now has an acronym – ORA. If this is associated with 'complete' RPE atrophy as well, which is defined as an area of RPE death of at least 250 microns in diameter, then the jazzy new term is cRORA, or complete RPE and outer retinal atrophy. This is new terminology for what we previously called GA. If there is atrophy of the outer retina and some RPE but smaller in nature and not as bad, this is termed 'incomplete' RORA, or iRORA, and can be understood as a form of 'pre-GA' atrophy. Keeping up with the shibboleths is the mark of a modern clinician.

Adult vitelliform macular dystrophy is a specific form of dry AMD where a symmetrical mound of subretinal subfoveal material occurs for many and varied reasons,

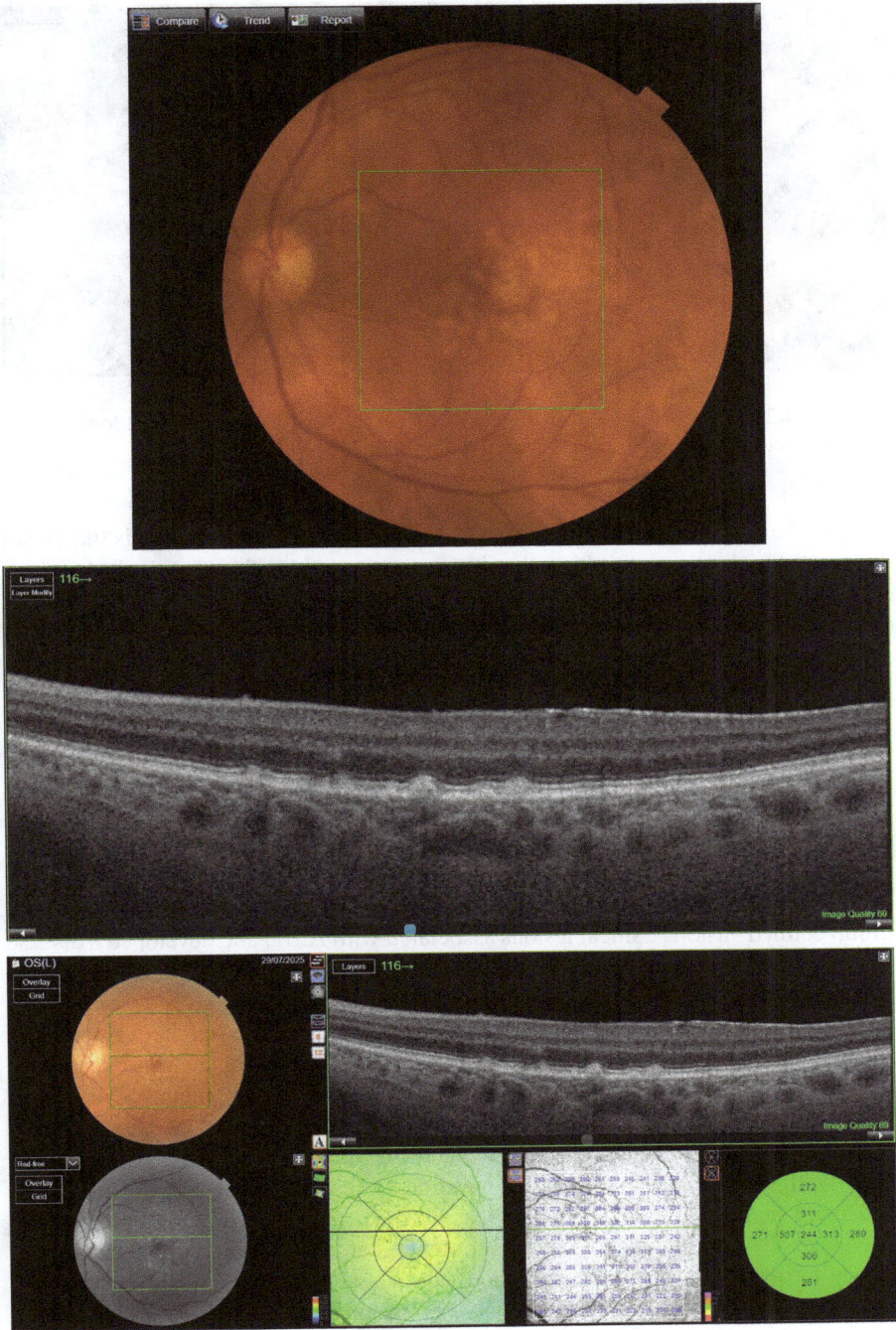

FIGURE 3.1 Drusen.

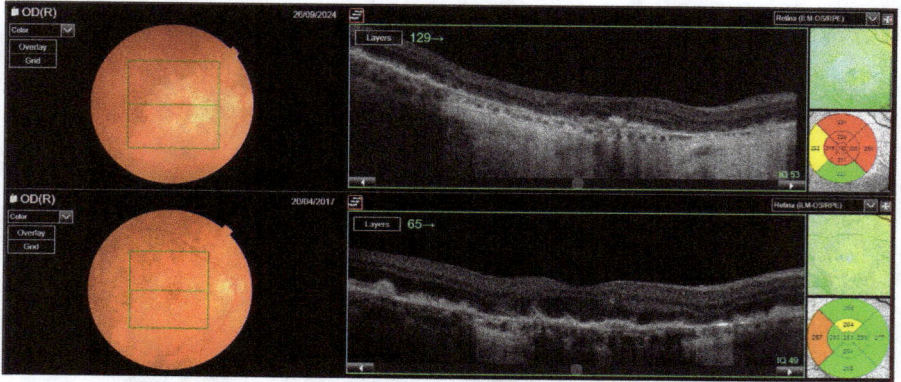

FIGURE 3.2 The growth of areas of geographic atrophy (GA) over time. The lower image was acquired in 2017 and the upper image acquired in 2024

none of them properly understood; the most important thing about this is that it can confuse clinicians into thinking that it represents neovascular change. It does not, although the picture becomes even more confused once resorption of this mound takes place because the partially reabsorbed vitelliform does resemble a fibrovascular pigment epithelial detachment (PED), though of course that would be sub-RPE rather than subretinal. Figure 3.3 displays an adult vitelliform lesion on an OCT scan.

Christiana Says...

In the practice of medicine, categorising the stages of disease is crucial because it provides a standardised way of describing the extent and severity of the disease, which helps our understanding of progression, treatment planning, prognosis and research into disease-modifying therapies. Staging diseases helps deepen our understanding. In 1995, the international age-related maculopathy epidemiological study group defined various clinical lesions associated with AMD and developed a disease severity grading system based largely on colour fundus photographs (CFPs), which was the main modality at that time (1).

Later on, the Stephen J. Ryan Initiative for Macular Research (formerly the Beckman Initiative for Macular Research) devised the Beckman classification, a widely accepted system to categorise the stages of dry AMD. Table 3.1 illustrates how this system works (2).

Since then, the introduction and evolution of multi-modal imaging, especially OCT, with widespread uptake has allowed depth-resolved assessment of the retina and more nuanced staging. With increasing research into GA, the non-exudative late-stage of AMD and identification of potential targets for intervention, it was necessary to devise standardized definitions and classifications for GA. Accordingly, the Classification of Atrophy meetings, a group of international experts in AMD, devised a consensus classification system based on OCT for GA (3). The consensus process involved evaluating the strengths and limitations of the various imaging modalities for GA and a recognition that each modality gives us insight and

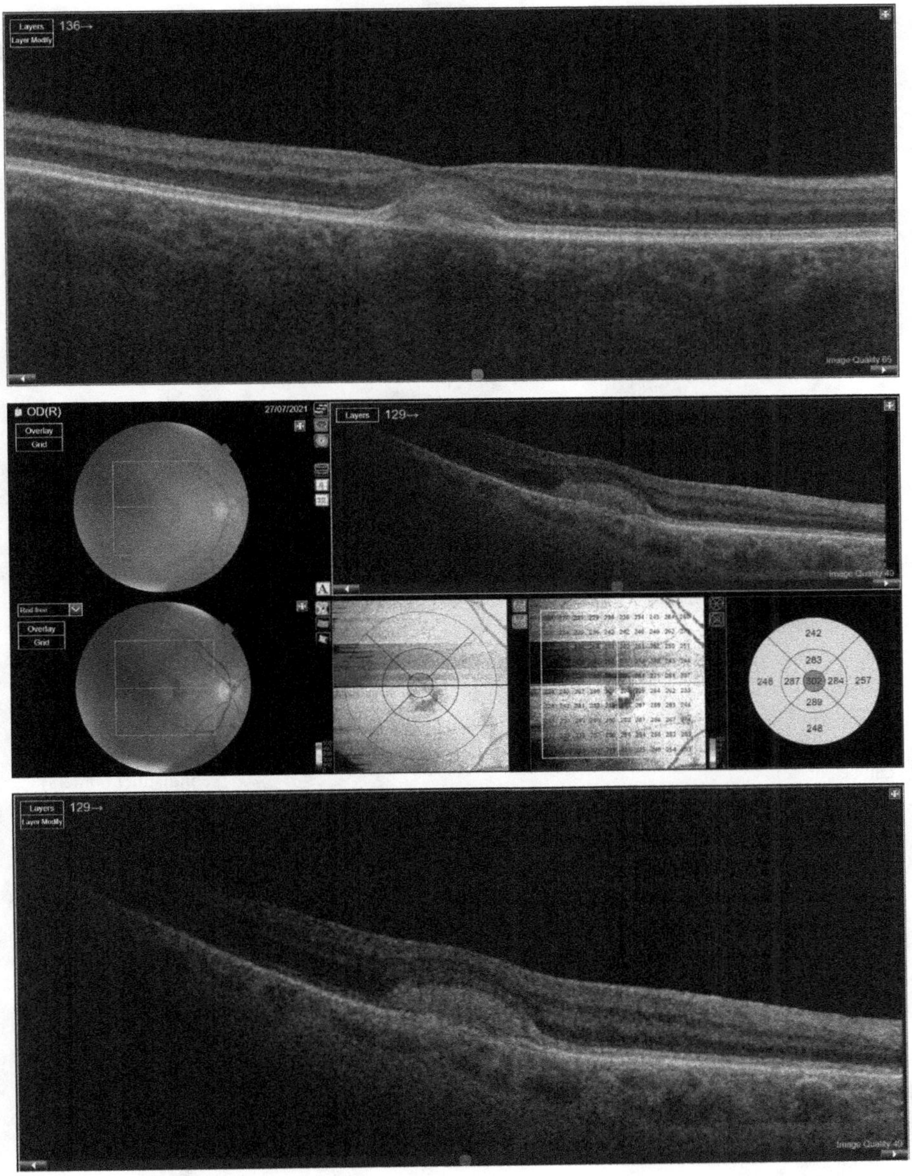

FIGURE 3.3   An OCT scan of an adult vitelliform lesion.

perspective that builds a more focused picture of the disease process. In particular, OCT allows depth-resolved resolution such that each retinal and choroidal layer can be reviewed and the severity of attenuation assessed, allowing identification of precursor lesions and early stages before the disease is detected as atrophy on CFP or fundus autofluorescence (FAF) (Table 3.2).

TABLE 3.1
The Beckman Classification System

Stage	Definition	Key Features
No AMD	No signs of AMD	No Drusen or only small drusen (<63 microns) and no pigmentary abnormalities
Early AMD	Low risk of progression	Presence of medium drusen (63–125 microns) without pigmentary abnormalities
Intermediate AMD	Moderate risk of progression	Large drusen (>125 microns) or medium drusen with RPE abnormalities
Late AMD	Vision loss likely	GA not involving the foveal centre or GA involving the foveal centre

TABLE 3.2
Demonstrates the Attributes of GA on Each Imaging Modality. (Modified from CAM Paper)

CFP	FAF	OCT	NIR
Sharply demarcated borders (contrast between GA and surrounding retina can be subtle)	Well-demarcated border (involvement of fovea may be difficult to assess)	Zone of hypertransmission of ≥250 μm	Well-demarcated borders (some eyes have isoreflective lesions resulting in indistinct borders)
Hypopigmentation	Hypoautofluorescence – black area similar to optic nerve head	Zone of attenuation or disruption of RPE ≥ 250 μm	Hyperreflective
Increased visibility of choroidal vessels	Diameter ≥ 250 μm	Evidence of overlying photoreceptor degeneration whose features include outer nuclear layer thinning, external limiting membrane loss and ellipsoid zone or interdigitation zone loss	Diameter ≥ 250 μm

RISK FACTORS

There are risk factors you can do something about and those that are unchangeable. The biggest, most well-known risk factor is, of course, smoking. **Smoking** causes everything and cigarette packets in the United Kingdom have, among a collection of off-putting images on their sides, an eye held open by a speculum accompanied by the ominous message 'smoking causes blindness'. Whilst ageing is of course the single biggest risk factor, hence the name of the condition, European ancestry or **genetic** predisposition is also important, but none of these are of course modifiable.

Smoking is by far the biggest modifiable risk factor and on average causes advanced AMF to occur 6 years earlier than would otherwise be the case. Giving up smoking is by far the most important thing a concerned patient can do.

Diet is also important. The basis of the AREDS 1 and 2 studies was to assess whether certain vitamins and minerals alter the progress of the condition. Though Christiana will discuss this further below, the long and short of it is that whilst the supplementation did, in fact, reduce progression rates marginally, the effect was only really significant in the group that had a poor diet with respect to broad-leaf green vegetables and so on. The cruel truth is that the group of patients most likely to go out of their way to access AREDS supplementation for the specific purpose of reducing the risk of progression are generally health conscious enough that they have good diets anyway, and are therefore the most unlikely to derive any benefit. The reverse is also true in a catch-22 situation. **Obesity** and **hypertension** are also risk factors, the reversal of which would be generally beneficial for multiple bodily systems.

HIGH-RISK DRY AGE-RELATED MACULAR DEGENERATION

There are many different risk stratification systems in existence for scoring dry AMD biomarker severity to predict the chance of progressing to advanced disease within a certain timeframe, with advanced disease being either GA or the development of neovascular AMD. Evidence for the validity of one over the other can be argued, but a few key principles hold fast that are worth bearing in mind here.

First, eyes with large drusen present a higher risk of progression than intermediate drusen and intermediate drusen present a higher risk than small drusen. A drusenoid PED presents an especially high risk. Figure 3.4 demonstrates an OCT image of a drusenoid PED.

Second, eyes with pigment changes at the macula present higher risk of progression than those without, with increased pigment disruption correlating with increased risk.

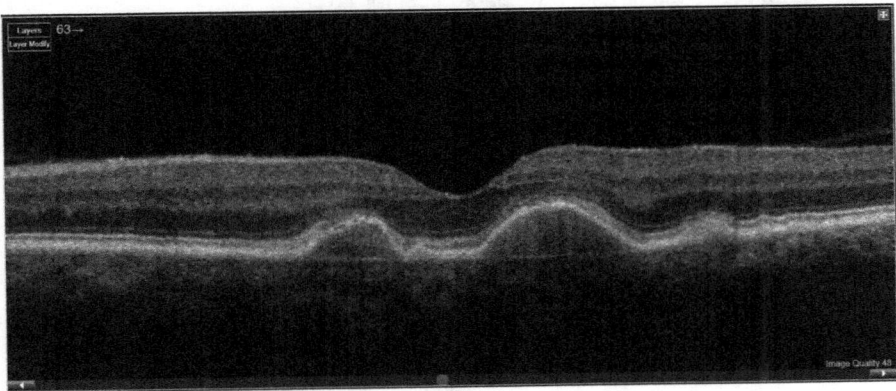

FIGURE 3.4   A drusenoid pigment epithelial detachment (PED).

Third, patients in which one eye has already progressed to advanced macular disease are more at risk of the same thing happening in the other eye than those without this progression. 'Both eyes are roughly the same age!' we tell our patients with a chuckle.

Christiana Says...

In science, we categorise levels of scientific evidence to help us determine how much weight to give the various sources of information we receive when making decisions. The strongest level of evidence (Level I) is evidence from systematic reviews of randomised controlled trials (RCTs). This is basically a synthesis of results from multiple high-quality studies, making this the gold standard. A systematic review of risk factors for progressing from intermediate AMD to advanced AMD (wet AMD or GA) confirmed that baseline drusen volume/size (the presence of large drusen ≥250 μm and increasing drusen volume) was associated with progression to neovascular AMD and photoreceptor layer thinning was associated with progression to GA (4). Other features such as focal hyperpigmentation, hyperreflective foci on OCT and reflectivity of drusen sub-structure have also been linked to progression to late-stage AMD but require further study to better quantify.

DIAGNOSIS

The most important thing here is making sure that 'dry' AMD is, in fact, dry and not 'wet'. The second thing to consider is that it isn't genetic in the sense of an inherited macular or retinal dystrophy. There are other differential diagnoses down the list, such as punctate inner choroidopathy (PIC), macular telangiectasia and such, but let us approach this in a stepwise manner:

Step 1: Is it AMD? Look for drusen in both eyes and/or hypo/hyperpigmentation of the RPE.

Step 1a: Is it neovascular (wet) AMD? Is there haemorrhage and/or exudate on fundoscopy or loss of retinal transparency? Are there hyporeflective spaces within the retina or under the photoreceptor layer?

Step 1b: Is it advanced dry AMD (GA)? Is there a sharply demarcated round or oval area of hypopigmentation with increased visibility of underlying choroidal vessels, or hypertransmission on OCT with abrupt cessation of RPE on either side and loss of the photoreceptor layer?

Step 2: If not, is it an inherited retinal dystrophy?

Step 3: If not, could it be due to a rarer cause? Is the patient atypical in any way?

Starting at the first step, any patient presenting with vision loss needs a careful history. Is it sudden or gradual? Gradual is more likely non-neovascular, of course. How long has the problem been present? If the problem exists a very long time, the vision is more likely to be worse. Are they aged? Do they have risk factors as mentioned above? A visual acuity needs to be taken as if the situation is critical, say 1.20 LogMAR or worse; then detailed investigations to differentiate the condition from

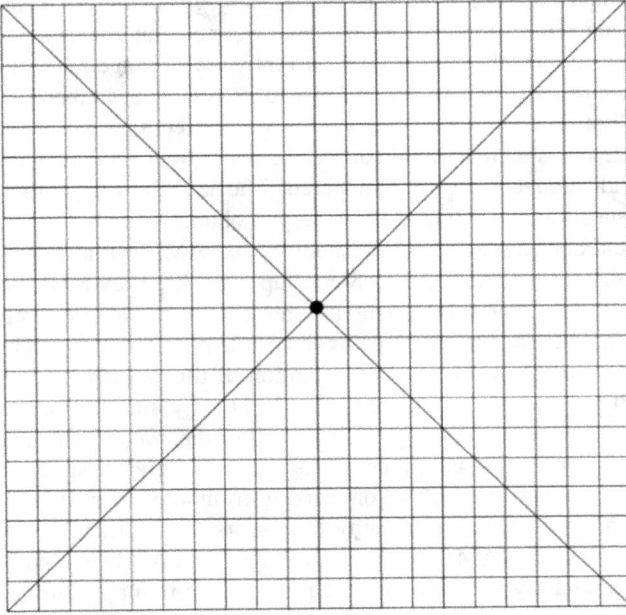

FIGURE 3.5   An Amsler chart.

neovascular AMD might well be purposeless because no treatment would be offered anyway. We treat the patient, not the condition. Is there distortion on Amsler grid testing? Amsler grids are sheets of graph paper with a dot in the middle. Patients close one eye and hold the grid approximately 30 cms away from the eye being tested and fixate on the dot, specifically looking for distortion of the straight lines, which can indicate early neovascular change. Figure 3.5 shows a typical Amsler chart. There are other Amsler chart variants, red on black and so on, but for all intents and purposes, they are only good to know for exam purposes and for research. In reality, even the typical Amsler grid isn't that good a tool for detecting early neovascular changes, but we hand them out to patients with dry AMD to self-monitor at home, along with a patient leaflet on AMD and perhaps some advice about modifiable risk factors such as smoking, mainly so we don't feel quite as impotent as we actually are in tackling a condition over which we have largely no control.

After dilating drops are instilled, the OCT scan is taken, which is by far the most valuable step in the diagnostic pathway. Oftentimes, we clinicians look at the OCT in detail and know what we will do and what we will tell the patient before we have even called their name, let alone looked at their fundus through the slit lamp. Simply put, we look for the presence of drusen, RPE changes such as atrophy or pigment migration, the absence of subretinal or intraretinal fluid and the absence of any obvious haemorrhage. The presence of these could well indicate 'wet' or neovascular AMD.

The slit lamp is a piece of theatre that usually gives context to the patient but does not add much to differentiating dry from wet macular changes. Do they have a cataract? If so, perhaps the poor vision, currently out of range for treatment, can be brought back into range where the cataract to be removed. Is there any peripheral retinal issue, not seen in the OCT scan, that could affect treatment? Is there a trabeculectomy bleb present that could put serious restrictions on where any intravitreal injection, if indicated, could be administered? The act of looking at the macula itself is simply no substitute for the level of detail you obtain with OCT.

If the patient does not have signs of neovascular AMD but is atypical for simple non-neovascular, or dry AMD, then Step 2 applies. Are they a bit young? Does it not look quite right? Then think about an inherited cause. Inherited retinal/macular dystrophies vie with diabetic retinopathy for prime place amongst sight-threatening conditions affecting the working-age population. If this is suspected, then ask for a detailed family history and consider electrophysiology and genetic testing to look for mutations. If there is no family history at all or the condition does not look like a genetic condition – say it is unilateral, for example – then consider a rarer cause such as macular telangiectasia, PIC or scarring from another disease process. Very rare causes can include solar retinopathy, laser scars and the like. However, common things are common; dry AMD accounts for 90% of all AMD and gets us all in the end, so by far and away the most important thing here is simply ruling out its more dangerous neovascular twin. Fundus fluorescein angiography (FFA) and/or indocyanine green angiography (ICGA) don't really have a role in diagnosing suspected dry AMD, though FAF is indeed useful in demonstrating areas of atrophy and quantifying the degree of affected macula.

Christiana Says...

GA is peculiar in that it most commonly starts in the extrafoveal region and expands circumferentially before finally involving the fovea in the later stages. As such, best corrected visual acuity (BCVA) is often not a good measure of the severity of GA or the impact on the patient. In fact, many people with intermediate AMD, and more so those progressing to GA, complain of difficulty recognising objects and navigating the world in dim lighting, difficulty reading especially low-contrast print and difficulty recognising faces and facial expressions. Yet, they may have 'good BCVA', even 0.00 LogMAR (6/6). Studies have investigated and confirmed that BCVA does not correlate with GA lesion size or progression (5). So the patient may be suffering worsening symptoms, but the way we measure their function in clinic does not reflect this. As clinicians, we are taught to start with a thorough history, which is even more important in a condition like GA as we enter an era where treatment may become available.

With more work in this area, other measures of visual function have been shown to correlate better with structural progression of GA on autofluorescence and OCT. These include low luminance visual acuity (LLVA), reading speed and contrast sensitivity function. LLVA is easy to perform in clinic because it is simply a modified version of BCVA typically using the same vision chart with a neutral density filter. It has been demonstrated that LLVA is reduced in early and intermediate AMD compared to control eyes, correlates with photoreceptor degeneration, and precedes deterioration of BCVA and is thus predictive of impending loss of foveal function (6, 7).

LLVA can be a very noisy test though, changing significantly from visit to visit, so more work is required to validate and standardize it's use in research and clinic. Of course, we can just ask the patient. Patient-reported outcome measures (PROMs) are a rigorous way of trying to do this in a scientifically reproducible way.

PROMs are validated questionnaires that assess health outcomes reported by patients. Several PROMs have been validated in AMD, and in particular GA. The most commonly used PROM in ophthalmology is the NEI-VFQ 25, which has been shown to be driven by the better eye, as would be expected. The VILL-33 has also been validated in early and intermediate AMD. The Functional Reading Index is a PROM that comprises seven questions and was developed to capture the impact of GA on reading (8).

Gaining momentum as a reproducible tool to capture structure–function correlation is microperimetry. Microperimetry involves presenting light stimulation of gradually decreasing intensities in a pointwise fashion to precisely determine the retinal sensitivity of a specific point of the retina. This is a precise method of determining the functional impact of AMD; however, it requires purchase of the equipment, takes skill to perform and can take an extended amount of time depending on the ability of the patient to fixate. Tablet-based forms are being evaluated and are likely to improve the accessibility of this functional assessment. In summary, it is important to recognise that BCVA does not capture the impact of AMD on patients' daily living activities and there are more robust, accessible tools out there that can better inform us and help identify patients who need additional support.

MANAGEMENT

When a patient comes to see you with dry AMD, and you've ruled out all else, deciding what to do can be more nuanced than is thought. Some patients can be trusted to report problems or deterioration either to you or their local, appropriately trained optometrist. Those sensible patients can be furnished with an Amsler grid, advice leaflet and phone number and can monitor their condition at home. Some other patients for multiple myriad and varied reasons either don't monitor their health properly, can't be trusted to report any problems due to a misplaced sense of 'causing people bother' or have simply abrogated their own responsibilities regarding their health in favour of the state doing so instead. With those patients, it would still be a great shame to miss the development of neovascular AMD at a treatable stage and therefore high-risk dry AMD patients; those with multiple intermediate or large drusen, drusenoid PEDs or who have a disciform macular scar in the other eye may benefit from an extra visit or two at increasingly spaced intervals so that any change could potentially be caught early. Considering the very limited resources and capacity of hospital eyecare services, this sort of condition might be ideal for medical retina qualified optometrists to monitor in the community, though healthcare economics would, of course, have to be worked out appropriately. Third-sector organisations such as the Royal National Institute for the Blind (RNIB) and Macular Society have a role to play in education as well, as do government organisations and society at large.

Patients will ask about various vitamin and mineral combinations that can be purchased over the counter, though these are not usually cheap and cannot be prescribed in most places. As doctors, we are always very reluctant to admit that 'nothing can be done', so oftentimes we are tempted to shrug embarrassingly if the patient asks about these tablets though we know the truth is that those who would be most willing to buy and take them are also those who would benefit the least. There is nothing wrong with making recommendations about diet, smoking and exercise, of course. All of these are important.

The new excitement with complement inhibitor injections, such as the recent hype with pegcetacoplan or avacincaptad pegol, has turned into a bit of a damp squib, unfortunately, following issues with licensing these medications outside of America. The arguments centre on a lack of visual improvement, risk of complications and the cost to both patients and healthcare systems. It is not for this book to pass judgement on the rightness or wrongness of these decisions except to be aware, if patients ask, that there is a treatment, but there is no access to it on this side of the Atlantic. It is important to understand the papers here, and this can be properly understood in the Christiana Says text below.

Some ophthalmologists advocate lens surgery to implant telescopic lenses to increase magnification at the expense of field of vision. These carry numerous risks and are not recommended for routine use for multiple reasons. In the past, it was observed that 'tickling' the drusen with Argon laser could cause them to disappear on occasion, though when it was realised that this did not translate to good vision and in effect simply accelerated the process toward a collapse into atrophy, the whole thing was abandoned. There are also far riskier surgical procedures performed such as macular translocation surgery, patch grafts of donor site RPE under the macula or stem cell therapy. Despite what the *Daily Mail* clippings your patients bring in might imply, these procedures are for research purposes only.

Visual rehabilitation is key. Dry macular degeneration is the cause of more certificates of visual impairment (CVI) being issued than any other condition by far, with over a quarter of all registrations being down to this condition alone. You would do your patient a far greater service by admitting that there is no practical treatment, and that counselling, psychological and practical support, managing with poor sight and planning for future deterioration is the best way forward. If the visual criteria are met, then filling in a CVI and involving local visual rehabilitation services with third-sector support can make a big difference to a patient's overall happiness and ability to function in the world, far more than any unevidenced recommendation about expensive over-the-counter tablets.

Christiana Says...

There is currently no intervention for intermediate AMD, although intervention at this stage would be desirable to prevent atrophy. The MACUSTAR project is a major European public-private research initiative focused on intermediate AMD, with the hope of developing interventions/new therapies at this stage (9). It includes a cross-sectional phase with four groups of patients with no AMD, early AMD, intermediate AMD and late AMD, and a longitudinal phase with functional, structural and PROMs with the promise of outcomes for regulatory and trial design use. The hope is that identifying and validating appropriate clinical endpoints will enable smaller, shorter, better-targeted studies that may accelerate dry AMD treatment development.

In the meantime, the U.S. Food and Drug Administration (FDA) recently approved a new treatment modality known as photobiomodulation as a treatment for intermediate AMD. Photobiomodulation uses low-level visible and near-infrared light to stimulate mitochondrial function in retinal cells. It is thought to work by increasing ATP production, reducing oxidative stress and inflammation, and supporting RPE and photoreceptor health. The Lightsite III study, the largest RCT with this modality to date, reported a 6 ETDRS letter improvement versus sham and GA incidence rate of 6.8% in treated eyes versus 24% in sham (10). These results are very promising. However, there are still questions about reproducibility due to some confounders in the trial design and reporting. Larger studies are likely to be undertaken in the United Kingdom before widespread uptake in the National Health Service (NHS), although this treatment is available privately.

There are many pathways implicated in GA, including lipid metabolism, mitochondrial pathways, complement pathway, extracellular matrix pathways and chronic inflammation. Of these, the complement pathway is the most extensively studied and evaluated. The complement pathway comprises a group of proteins that circulate in the blood and tissues and act as a first line of defence against pathogens/invaders to recognise and destroy them to prevent illness or injury. In AMD, the complement system is inappropriately activated, resulting in increased inflammation, formation of drusen and cell death. There is genetic evidence from genome-wide association studies (GWASs), identification of complement proteins in drusen and GA tissues, and preclinical studies showing the role of complement dysfunction in GA-like pathology. In February 2023, the FDA approved pegcetacoplan (Syfovre), a C3 and C3b inhibitor, delivered by intravitreal injection monthly or every other month, for the management of GA. This was based on two global parallel double-blind RCTs, OAKS and DERBY, which showed that pegcetacoplan reduced anatomical progression of GA by up to 21% at 24 months (11, 12).

In August 2023, avacincaptad pegol, a complement factor C5 inhibitor, was also approved by the FDA after the GATHER2 global RCT demonstrated up to 19% reduction in GA lesion growth compared to sham. However, neither treatment demonstrated a beneficial impact on functional endpoints by 24 months including BCVA, LLVA, reading speed and microperimetry. In addition, both treatments were associated with increased conversion to wet AMD compared to sham, incidence of intraocular inflammation and even rare cases of occlusive vasculitis reported in the real-world studies. As such, whilst the FDA-approved pegcetacoplan is based on reduction in anatomical progression, the European Medicines Agency (EMA) and Medicines and Healthcare products Regulatory Agency (MHRA) did not agree that the risk outweighed the benefit, especially because no prespecified functional benefit was demonstrated (Table 3.3).

More recently, a post hoc analysis of the AREDS and AREDS2 trials reported a significant reduction in progression of non-foveal GA to the fovea with oral nutrient supplementation, suggesting that the formulation may augment the natural phenomenon of foveal sparing seen in GA (13). Pending confirmatory trials, this suggests there may be some benefit to those over-the-counter pills after all!

In summary, GA remains a significant unmet need with public health consequences. At present, we can offer listening ears, support through eye clinic liaison officers and our patient charities, and hope in the form of clinical trials investigating promising candidates that may one day slow, halt or reverse GA.

TABLE 3.3
Summary of Landmark Clinical Trials of Complement Inhibitors in Geographic Atrophy

	Intervention	Comparator	No. of Participants	Eligible Participants	Primary Endpoint	Primary Outcome	Importance and Practice Implication
DERBY/OAKS	Pegcetacoplan (Syfovre) • Monthly or • Every other month	Sham • Monthly or • Every other month	1258	Key inclusion: • Age: ≥60 • BCVA 6/96 or better • Foveal involvement allowed • Fellow eye choroidal neovascular membrane (CNVM) allowed	Change in total area of GA at 12 months on FAF	Monthly arm: Reduced GA growth by 21% at 12 months in OAK (12% in DERBY) Every other month arm: Reduced GA growth by 16% at 12 months in OAK (11% in DERBY)	Proved for the first time that complement inhibition can slow GA progression rate. Functional benefit not demonstrated in prespecified randomised cohort
GATHER2	Monthly 2 mg Avacincaptad pegol (Izervay) • At month 12, patients receiving monthly Izervay were re-randomised 1:1 to monthly or every other month ACP 2 mg	Sham	448	Key inclusion criteria: Age: ≥50 Non-centre-involving GA	Mean rate of change in GA lesion area over 12 months on FAF	18% reduction in GA growth at 12 months in monthly	Confirms the role of complement inhibition in slowing GA growth. Did not demonstrate prespecified functional benefit

REFERENCES

1. Bird AC et al. An international classification and grading system for age-related maculopathy and age-related macular degeneration. Surv Ophthalmol. 1995; 39(5):367–374.
2. Ferris FL et al. Clinical classification of age-related macular degeneration. Ophthalmology. 2013; 120(4):844–851.
3. Sadda SR et al. Consensus definition for atrophy associated with age-related macular degeneration on OCT: Classification of atrophy report 3. Ophthalmology. 2018; 125(4):537–548.
4. Hagag AM et al. Systematic review of prognostic factors associated with progression to late-age-related macular degeneration: Pinnacle study report 2. Surv Ophthalmol. 2024; 69 (2):165–172.
5. Heier JS, Pieramici D, Chakravarthy U, Patel SS, Gupta S, Lotery A, Lad EM, Silverman D, Henry EC, Anderesi M, Tschosik EA, Gray S, Ferrara D, Guymer R; Chroma and Spectri Study Investigators. Visual function decline resulting from geographic atrophy: Results from the Chroma and Spectri phase 3 trials. Ophthalmol Retina. 2020; 4:673–688. https://doi.org/10.1016/j.oret.2020.01.019
6. Abidi M, Karrer E, Csaky K, Handa JT. A clinical and preclinical assessment of clinical trials for dry age-related macular degeneration. Ophthalmol Sci. 2022; 2:100213. https://doi.org/10.1016/j.xops.2022.100213
7. Balaskas K, Glinton S, Keenan TDL, Faes L, Liefers B, Zhang G, Pontikos N, Struyven R, Wagner SK, McKeown A, Patel PJ, Keane PA, Fu DJ. Prediction of visual function from automatically quantified optical coherence tomography biomarkers in patients with geographic atrophy using machine learning. Sci Rep. 2022; 12:15565. https://doi.org/10.1038/s41598-022-19413-z.
8. Kimel M et al. Functional reading independence index: A new patient-reported outcome measure for patients with geographic atrophy. Invest Ophthalmol Vis Sci. 2016; 57:6298–6304.
9. Finger RP et al. MACUSTAR: development and clinical validation of functional, structural and patient-reported endpoints in intermediate age-related macular degeneration. Ophthalmologica. 2019; 241(2):61–72.
10. Boyer D et al. Lightsite III: 13-month efficacy and safety evaluation of multiwavelength photobiomodulation in nonexudative (dry) age-related macular degeneration using the Lumithera Valeda Light Delivery System. Retina. 2024; 44(3):487–497.
11. Heier JS et al. Pegcetacoplan for the treatment of geographic atrophy secondary to age-related macular degeneration (OAKS and DERBY): Two multicentre, randomised, double-masked, sham-controlled, phase 3 trials. Lancet. 2023; 402(10411):1434–1448.
12. Khanani A et al. Efficacy and safety of avacincaptad pegol in patients with geographic atrophy (GATHER2): 12-month results from a randomised, double-masked, phase 3 trial. Lancet. 2023; 402(10411):1449–1458.
13. Keenan TDL et al. Oral antioxidant and lutein/zeaxanthin supplements slow geographic atrophy progression to the fovea in age-related macular degeneration. Ophthalmology. 2025; 132(1):14–29.

4 Neovascular Age-Related Macular Degeneration

There are many names by which this condition is known – wet, exudative, neovascular and many more. 'Wet' is particularly confusing for patients because they then conflate their watery eyes with age-related macular degeneration (AMD), and opportunities for misunderstandings abound. Likewise, neovascular can be confused with 'new vessel' development in ischaemic conditions such as diabetes or retinal vein occlusion (RVO), but because it is the superior term here and the pathophysiology *is* sort of the same, this is the term we will preferentially use here. In taking notes, 'neovascular AMD' is often shortened as nAMD.

WHAT IS 'WET' AGE-RELATED MACULAR DEGENERATION?

Wet, or neovascular AMD, is a complication of dry, or non-neovascular AMD. Ischaemic cells at the macula are made ischaemic by deteriorating retinal pigment epithelium (RPE) and the deposition of waste material in the form of drusen under the retina. These conditions cause issues with the delivery of oxygen and other nutrients from the choriocapillaris of the choroid to the avascular outer retinal layers, which are otherwise dependent on efficient transfer to survive. Those cells in danger have a choice; die or call for help. If they chemically call for help, this usually involves releasing growth factors, by far the most important and famous of which is vascular endothelial growth factor (VEGF). There are many others, such as platelet-derived growth factor and angiopoietin-2 (Ang-2), that also play some sort of role, though that role is not that well understood at present. Similarly, there is not just one VEGF. Like a large Catholic family, there are many siblings, cousins and uncles, such as VEGFA, VEGFB, and VEGFC, and even within each of these there are isoforms such as VEGFA121, VEGFA145 and VEGFA165 until before long we are bewildered and confused. The exact details may or may not be interesting, but they are not for us clinicians.

What are the results of this growth factor soup? As the name suggests, vascular structures grow from an area with ample blood supply to the ischaemic area in the macula. On the face of it, this is good; after all, this is how healing tissues and growth generally occur almost everywhere else in the body. However, in reality, it is bad. It would have been much better had the body not attempted to solve this problem in this manner. The road to hell is paved with good intentions, and in the eye, for multiple reasons, the blood vessels that grow are of poor quality and lack direction, spilling their precious but toxic blood into the delicate internal structures of the retina causing scarring and permanent damage to vision. These new blood vessels grow much more commonly from the choroid, the second-most vascular structure in the human body after the carotid body, but a small number can grow additionally from the internal retinal circulation and form an anastomosis with the vessels growing up

36

DOI: 10.1201/9781003628309-4

from the choroid. An alternative name for the meshwork of vessels that grows in and under the retina is therefore the choroidal neovascular membrane (CNVM). Medical Retina loves its acronyms.

If the cells die instead, then no growth factor soup is released (dead men can't call for help) and the lesion progresses into atrophy.

CLASSIFICATION

In the old days, before the advent of OCT scans, when fundus fluorescein angiography (FFA) ruled the diagnostic roost, the first formal classification was divided into lesions. Cases in which you could obviously see the blood vessel complexes were called 'classic' lesions, whereas a sort of generalised leak of dye, where the blood vessel complex was not obvious, was called 'occult'. Occult, meaning 'hidden', such as in the occult arts, magic and so forth. This became a bit more complex if a lesion was a bit of both; they were called 'minimally classic' if they were obvious in less than half of the total area of leakage or 'predominantly classic' if the blood vessel complex was obvious in more than half. At the time, the treatment was photodynamic therapy (PDT), where verteporfin dye is injected into a vein while a diode laser is shone at the macula, specifically at the leaking complex. The choice to treat or not and how effective that treatment would be was directly correlated with the nature of the lesion itself. In those days, the specifics made a difference. Now they do not.

What made these lesions behave on angiography the way that they did? In short, the RPE. An intact RPE shields light, so if the neovascular complex is entirely located between Bruch's membrane and the RPE, the exact nature of the lesion defined by our ability to detect the dye in an FFA is difficult to ascertain due to the cloaking effect. This makes the leakage general and the CNVM complex occult (see Figure 4.1). If the membrane has grown through the RPE, then all the light emitted

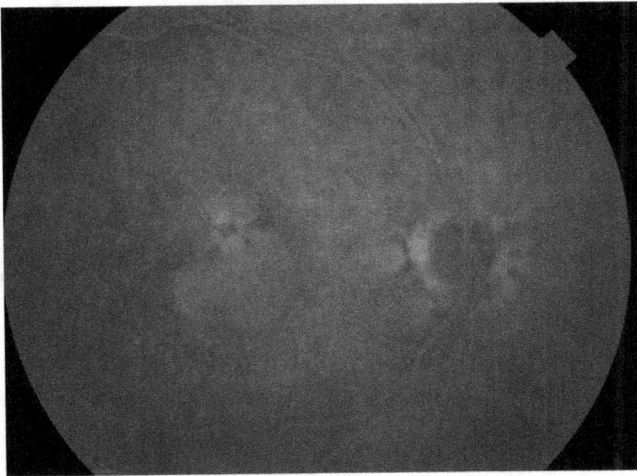

FIGURE 4.1   An occult choroidal neovascular membrane on fundus fluorescein angiogram (FFA).

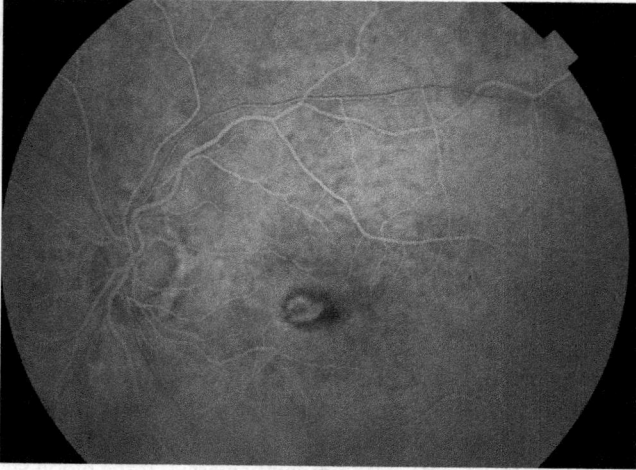

FIGURE 4.2 A classic choroidal neovascular membrane on FFA.

by the FFA process will be readily and greedily detected by the hungry angiogram machine, and sometimes beautiful branching lacy patterns are seen where the individual blood vessels and their anastomoses are obvious (see Figure 4.2). This is why classic membranes are not occult, though a more fitting term would be perhaps the antonym such as 'obvious', especially because occult membranes are more common than classic and therefore, in a way, more 'classic' than classic.

Blood vessel complexes that are partially under and partially over the RPE make up minimally and predominantly classic membranes, depending on the proportions of each. A third type, termed retinal angiomatous proliferation (RAP), which occurs when the blood vessel complex originates from the inner retinal circulation and develops mainly within the retina, as opposed to under it. The textbook-based classic descriptor for a RAP lesion is a 'hairpin bend' on indocyanine green angiography (ICGA) that occurs when the retinal and choroidal circulations anastomose in a sharp switchback loop. Even the term 'retinal angiomatous proliferation' is clumsy and simply means a growth of blood vessels in the retina. Happily, the advent of optical coherence tomography (OCT) and OCT angiography (OCT-A) meant a sweeping away of the old terms and a new way of describing lesions that was more sensible all a round.

The membranes are now divided into types 1, 2 and 3. Some people attempt to use a type 4, but this is simply a human response to simplicity in trying to overcomplicate things. It will only be a matter of time before someone tries to introduce a type 5 and 6, too. A far greater service is afforded your specialty by simplifying things rather than complicating matters. A **type 1 CNVM** is what used to be called occult, but is no longer properly occult because the OCT readily uncovers the complex in great detail. Whilst the RPE is usually snug up against Bruch's membrane, in the case of a type 1 membrane where a vascular complex is

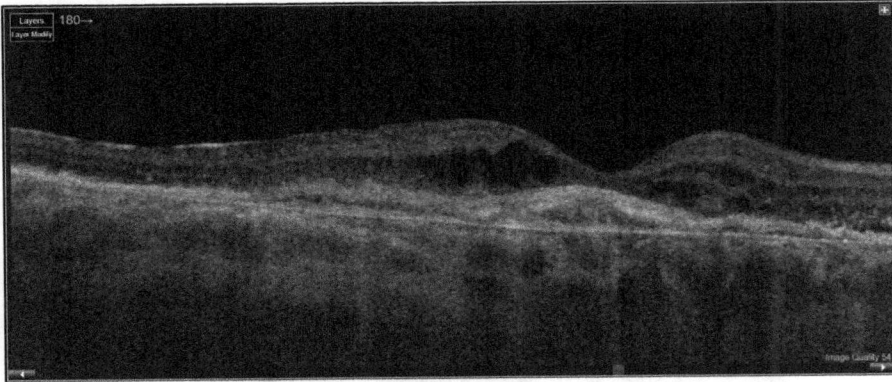

FIGURE 4.3 A type 1 membrane with double-layer sign.

stuck in between, there is a lifting off of the RPE that is usually shallow but wide. This can form the so-called double-layer sign because the RPE and Bruch's, usually together, are separated and apart and can look like slightly wonky train tracks (see Figure 4.3).

This is of course a form of pigment epithelial detachment (PED) and occurs on a spectrum. Whilst the most common manifestation is shallow and broad, the shallowness can blend into height and the broadness need not be so broad. As the PED increases in height, it can transition from fibrovascular on OCT to mixed, with layers of darker-coloured fibrovascular tissue intermingled with fluid to the PED being almost entirely fluid-filled – a so-called serous PED. Some longer-standing type 1 membranes can show signs of multilayered bands of fluid and membrane inside the epithelial detachment. A sign of activity is a prechoroidal cleft, a fluid-filled slit of fluid between Bruch's membrane and a band of CNVM tissue above and inside the PED itself. The PED can show signs of being tethered or kinked in places, disrupting its symmetry and shape, with these areas being a result of the CNVM attaching itself to the RPE in an attempt to grow through it. Figure 4.4 highlights this effect. The PED may also be high and wide, which increases the risk of the RPE detaching from Bruch's (known as a rip). This can occur spontaneously or after intravitreal injections. The rate of RPE rip varies depending on case series reviewed, but in most trials tends to be between 1% and 3%. Visual outcome may still be good, especially if the rip does not involve the fovea. If an RPE rip is suspected, consider a high-density OCT scan and fundus autofluorescence, which will show an area of hypoautofluorescence, where the RPE is no longer present.

The sure-fire tell-tale piece of evidence that drives this diagnosis home is then provided by the OCT-A, where the slice through the suspicious area on the OCT reveals the presence of a nicely demarcated neovascular complex. Many authors have gone to the time and trouble of delineating exact types of membrane complexes depending on their shape; a Medusa head if the branches extend outward in a

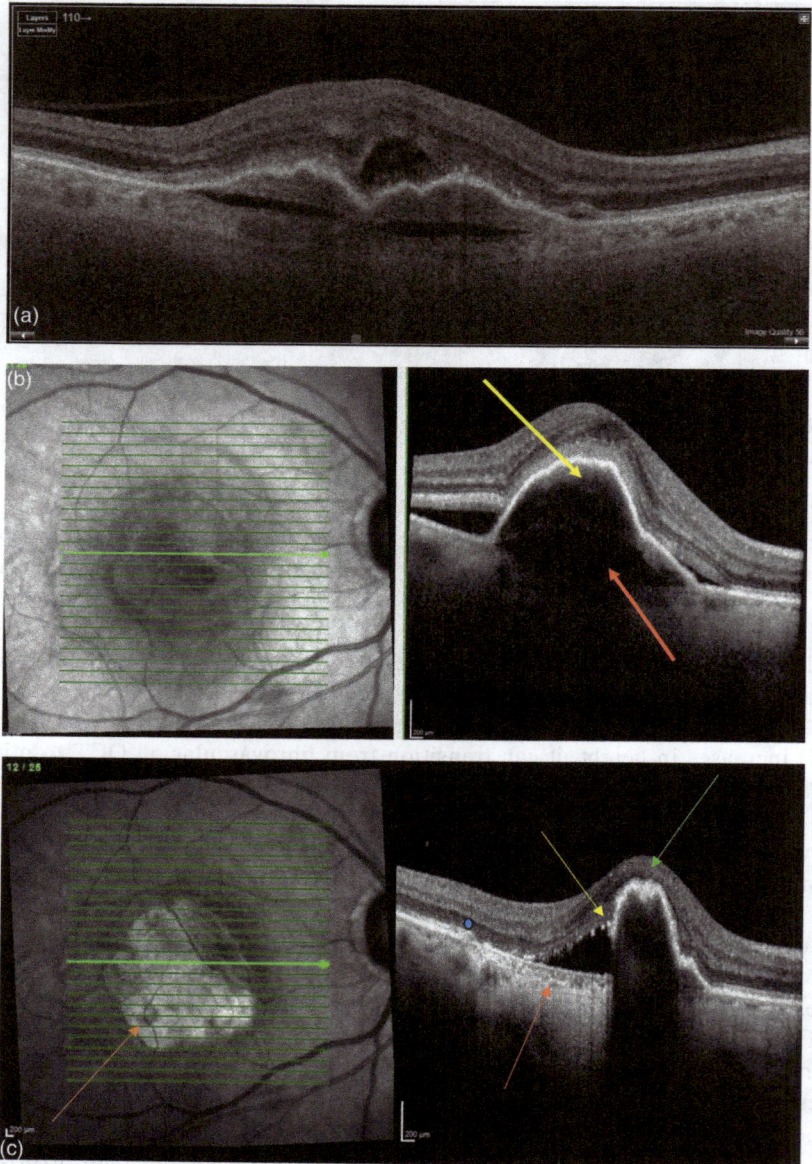

FIGURE 4.4 (a) A fibrovascular pigment epithelial detachment (PED) with kinking of the RPE due to tethering with CNVM. (b) Large mixed serous and fibrovascular PED. Yellow arrow: moderate reflectivity in sub-RPE space consistent with fibrovascular tissue. Red arrow: optically clear, hyporeflective area consistent with serous fluid. (c) RPE tear noted 1 month after intravitreal injection. Yellow arrow: discontinuity in RPE layer. Green arrow: irregular, rolled RPE edge. Red arow: area of bare Bruch's membrane and choroidal hypertransmission where the RPE is torn away. Blue dot: abrupt cessation of RPE. Orange arrow: Hyperreflectivity on near infrared denoting bare choroid. (d) Fundus autofluorescence denoting absence of RPE as area of hypoautofluorescence. *(Continued)*

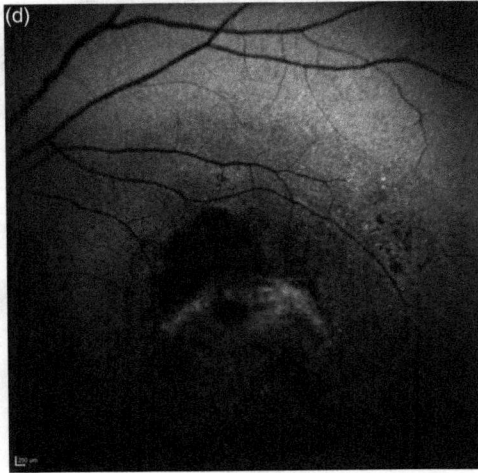

FIGURE 4.4 *(Continued)*

characteristic 'headful of snakes' manner (see Figure 4.5), a sea fan if the branches are predominantly organised facing and growing in one direction (see Figure 4.6), a 'dead tree' if the branches appear inactive, thin and brittle and many others. This is mainly medical ornithology again, and though coming up with these sorts of classifications are a way to further one's reputation and publish papers, it matters very little to the clinician toiling away at the coal face. You could just as easily classify membranes that look like ducks, swirls or merry-go-rounds. It doesn't help. What matters is whether a distinct membrane complex is present or not. If so, the second question to ask is whether it is active or not.

Measuring activity is what counts, and this is surprisingly simple, despite what countless papers and textbooks might have you believe. Is there any haemorrhage present due to the presence of the membrane (and not, say, diabetes)? If so, it is active. Is there any intraretinal fluid (IRF) present? If so, it is active. Lastly, is there any subretinal fluid (SRF) present? If so, you've guessed it, it's active. If there is a membrane present, but it is inactive, then this is vital for knowing whether to treat it (see below). Even the type of activity is important because the presence of SRF alone is much less damaging than either IRF or haemorrhage. But we are getting ahead of ourselves. Any fluid below the RPE is not considered 'activity' in the sense that treatment would be indicated. Anti-VEGF injections are not given for anything sub-RPE, despite what the big companies would have you believe.

A danger of classifying all sub-RPE membranes as type 1 is that a whole different form of membrane entity, **polypoidal choroidal vascularisation** (PCV), is lumped in with this as well. These are more aggressive bleeding polypoidal blood vessels that typically have large or very large PEDs associated with them, which again can be notched, but typically are more likely to have SRF and less likely by far to have IRF. The degree of haemorrhage present is also usually a lot more pronounced. Indeed, the older name for this condition was 'posterior uveal bleeding syndrome'. But it

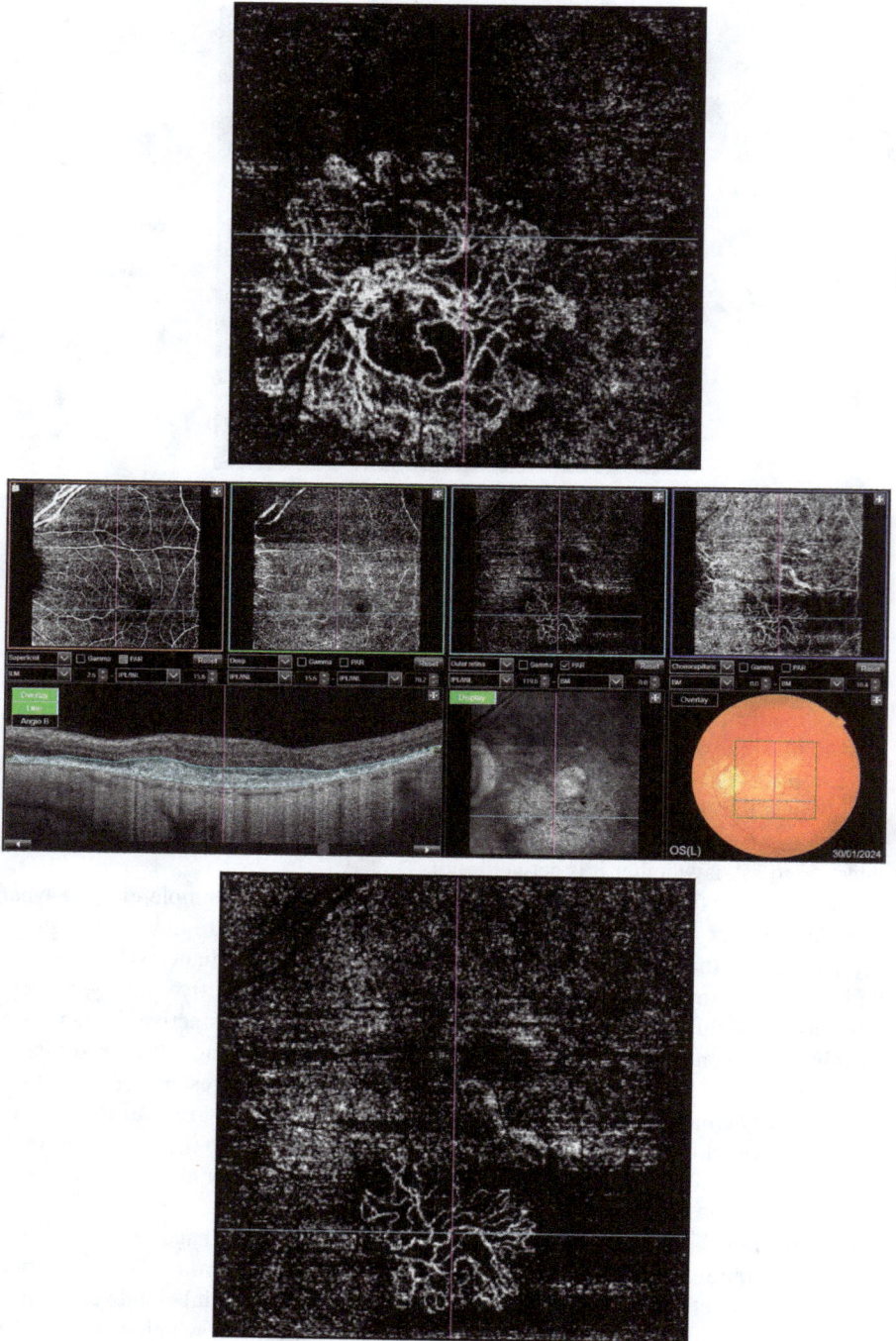

FIGURE 4.5 A Medusa head CNVM.

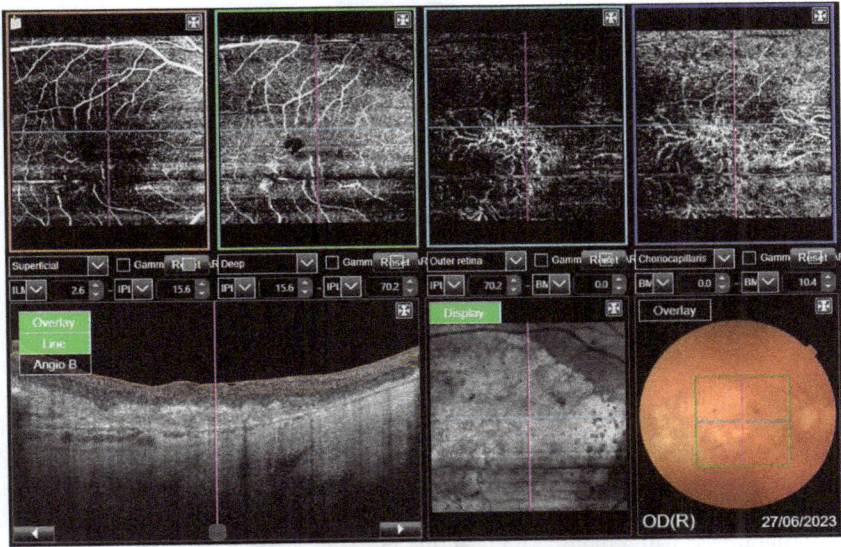

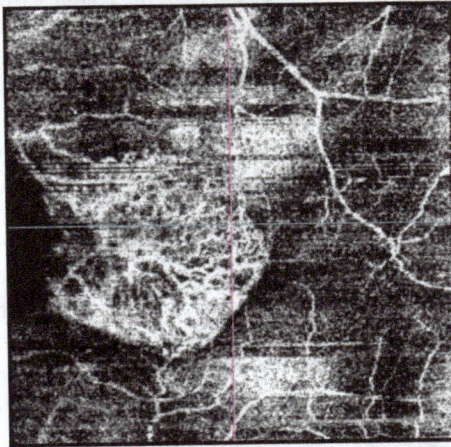

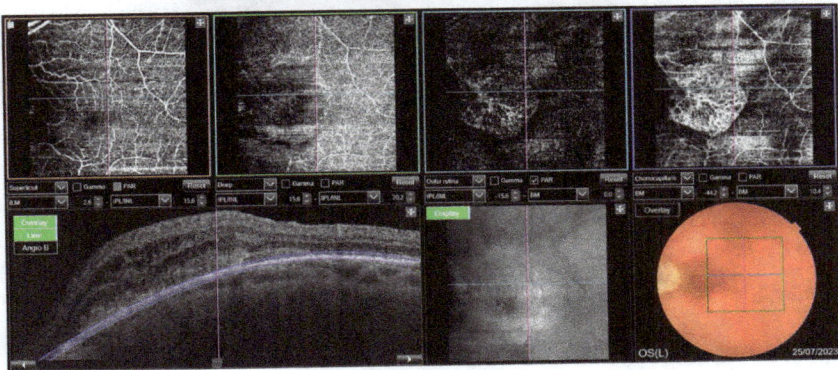

FIGURE 4.6 A sea fan-shaped CNVM.

doesn't matter, it really doesn't. The treatment is the same. Whether you accidentally classify a type 1 membrane as PCV or vice versa is immaterial. Gone are the days of PDT in the vast majority of cases. Certain people may point out that PDT is much better than injections at reducing the anatomical appearance of PCV versus a regular type 1 membrane, but as the visual outcomes are better for both with injections, so what? Don't stress too much over this distinction. Just be aware it exists.

A **type 2 CNVM** used to be called a classic membrane, where a portion of the neovascular membrane has grown through the RPE and is now subretinal. Whether it is minimally classic or predominantly classic is again immaterial; it is a type 2 membrane now. On clinical examination, compared with the very rarely bleeding type 1 membrane, a type 2 membrane is much more likely to bleed. A halo of blood sometimes appears around the growing edge of the complex or a spot here or there, rather than the catastrophic haemorrhaging you can see with PCV. OCT scans will reveal, in addition to type 1 CNVM signs, some changes between the RPE and the retina itself, in the subretinal space. This will usually be fibrovascular material between the two layers, with actively growing parts being 'fluffier' than the more mature stable parts that are more distinctly edged. The amount of IRF tends to be more pronounced if the membrane is active in comparison with type 1 CNVMs, as might be expected. The pathology is closer to the retina itself and as a consequence, there is generally greater visual disturbance and damage to the precious photoreceptor architecture. Figure 4.7 displays an OCT scan of a patient with type 2 CNVM with a fluffy border.

There will be a membrane present on OCT-A corresponding to this area, but again, making distinctions between types 1 and 2 by painstakingly poring over scans is unnecessary. The treatment is the same. It is largely a waste of our precious time. What *is* important is whether it is active or not, and determining this the same criteria as with a type 1 CNVM is applied – SRF, IRF or haemorrhage. It must be remembered that OCT-A will still demonstrate the presence of a membrane even if the membrane has been shut down by injections. People do say, of course, how the characteristics of an inactive membrane are different from an

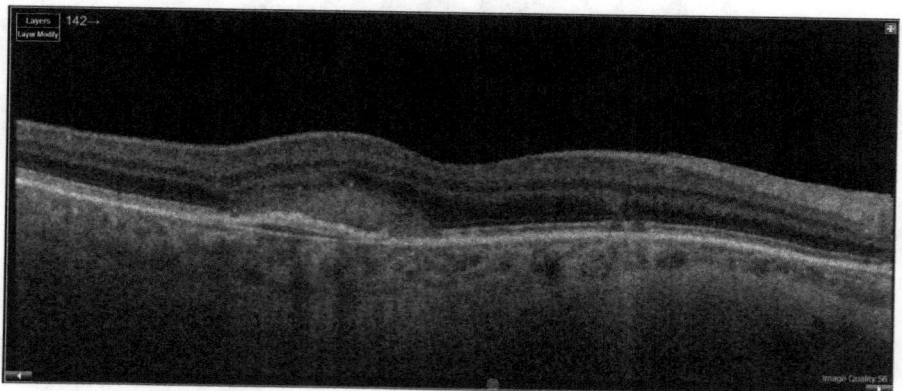

FIGURE 4.7   An OCT of a patient with type 2 CNVM with a 'fluffy border'.

active one, but this is a complex thing to decide and ultimately simply looking for signs of activity is by far the most useful thing that can be done. Instead of scrutinising a suspect for signs that he may be a murderous type, looking around him and behind him for murder victims is far easier and more useful. Older membranes scar down, termed gliosis, which is what scar tissue in the central nervous system is called because it is partly comprised of glial cells. Borders are distinct as well, instead of being fluffy.

What used to be called a RAP lesion is now a **type 3 CNVM** and presents much the same as the other subtypes. There is a slightly greater preponderance of small haemorrhages and some exudation, but the overlap is so small and the relevance so little that there isn't much usefulness in straining over specific distinctions here. OCT reveals more action in the retina itself, and as the condition progresses this extends down towards the choroid. The initial subclassifications of type 3 CNVMs, produced by that hero of Medical Retina John Donald Gass ('JD Gass'), is divided into stages 1, 2 and 3, depending on whether the membrane is restricted to the retina, has grown down into the subretinal space or reached the choroid, respectively. This is interesting insofar as it explains how things progress, but it is not useful clinically because all roads lead to Rome and the end destination is the same. So please don't stress too much over these specific classifications. Figure 4.8 displays an OCT image of a type 3 CNVM.

The last end-stage classification of note is the disciform macular scar. This is where most roads lead eventually if treatment is not instituted in a timely manner. This name is an overly complicated way of saying simply 'round scar at the macula' and is a combination of gliotic scarring and a spectrum of structural disturbances brought on by the effects of bleeding and exudation. Clinically, it appears as a whitish irregular scar at the macula, with the OCT displaying grossly distorted anatomy with large spaces and scar tissue extending in various directions. Perhaps OCT-A might reveal huge juicy vessel complexes with variable bits shut down, but the details are unimportant as nothing can be usefully done treatment-wise and the name of the game is support. An OCT of a disciform scar is displayed in Figure 4.9.

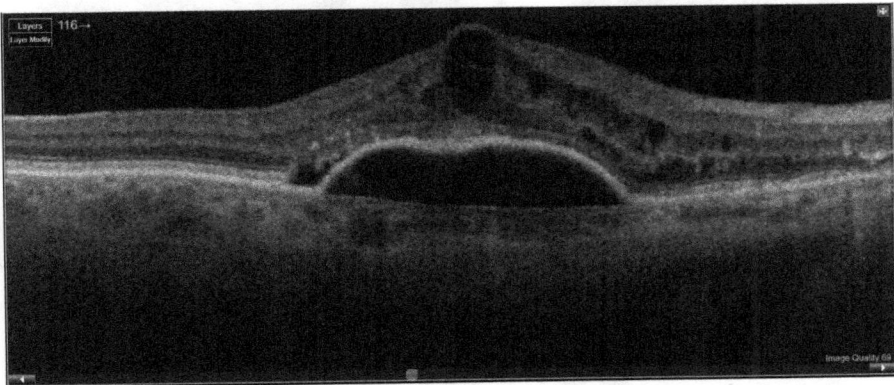

FIGURE 4.8 An OCT of a type 3 CNVM.

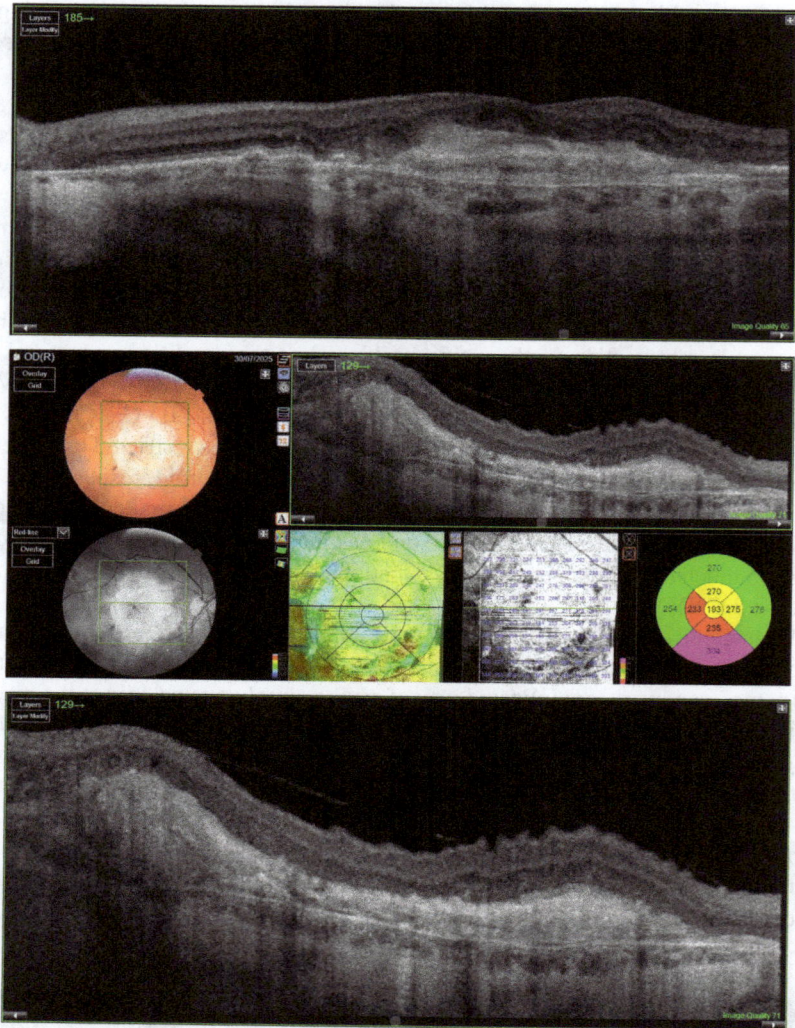

FIGURE 4.9   An OCT of a disciform macular scar.

NOMENCLATURE

It should be stated here that there are many terms bandied about that mean the same thing. CNVM is the same as nAMD, which is the same as the macular neovascular membrane (MNV), and perhaps by the time you are reading this another term will have been invented. They are all the same, though the theologians of our profession will doubtlessly try and painstakingly pick apart how they are not on points of obscure ideology, but to us simple clinicians, they are the same. Use whichever one you like, but don't make up any new terms, please!

Christiana Says...

I would argue that the details are interesting *and* useful for clinicians to know, especially in the age of AI, but we digress! On the topic of making up new terms, we do have to acknowledge that the advent of OCT-A has meant that we can now detect MNVMs that are not associated with any exudation. These non-exudative MNVMs have been shown to be present in up to 24% of fellow eyes of patients with unilateral exudative MNVM (1,2). They appear to be a precursor to conversion to exudative AMD, and it has been shown that the incidence of clinically evident exudation ranges between 20% and 80% during 6 months to 2 years of follow-up. At present, there appears to be no benefit from treating these lesions before they become exudative. In fact, there is a school of thought that they may be helpful in maintaining nourishment of the RPE and outer retina. The OCT-A demonstrates these lesions in detail, whilst OCT alludes to their presence when a shallow PED (known as a double-layer sign) is detected. However, as retinal imaging and research evolve, these lesions may well be one of the avenues by which we prevent nAMD, so it is worth keeping informed as knowledge in this area evolves.

RISK FACTORS

Without reinventing the wheel, these are broadly the same as the risk factors mentioned in Chapter 3, though there are a few added risks specifically for the development of neovascular membranes without them being specifically secondary to age-related factors. Basically, anything that damages the RPE/Bruch's complex can cause a secondary CNVM to grow through the defect, which can then bleed, leak and scar the macula. This could be due to damage as a result of chronic central serous chorioretinopathy (CSCR), laser scars administered for diabetic eye disease, degeneration secondary to choroidal lesions such as an osteoma, scarring as a result of uveitic conditions such as punctate inner choroidopathy (PIC); the list is basically endless. However, strictly speaking, if the development of the membrane is not due to age-related changes, it is **not** termed wet AMD, nAMD or any of the other epithets. It is termed a secondary CNVM, even though, in effect, nAMD is also secondary to something – ageing – and at the end of the day, the treatment is much the same anyway – injections (see below). So again, in a patient with an actively leaking membrane, straining your brain over whether it is truly age-related or secondary to some other process is not such a good use of your valuable time, unless that other condition warrants some sort of treatment in addition to that for the membrane.

HIGH-RISK LESIONS

Even though all roads do indeed lead to Rome, the pace of travel is variable and there are numerous inns and taverns to stay in along the way. Some variants of nAMD are more dangerous than others and lead to earlier destruction. There is, of course, wide overlap between how different membrane types behave, so we should absolutely refrain from saying 'type 1 CNVM membranes always need this, whilst type 2 need that', but as a general rule of thumb, PCV is haemorrhagically aggressive, type 3 is damaging to the retina and can be difficult to treat, type 2 is better than type 3 but still more damaging than type 1, and type 1 is the most benign but can still cause very serious visual problems.

Far better to stratify the risk of these membranes, and therefore treatment, based on the type of activity going on rather than the type of membrane. Bleeding of any kind is damaging and bad, and patients benefit the most from prompt and timely treatment. IRF, without the presence of blood, is also damaging, if not quite as damaging as blood itself, and again treatment is almost always indicated if the patient is agreeable. The presence of SRF, without the presence of IRF or blood, is a different animal.

The presence of a slip of SRF is a low-risk lesion by itself. It is still active, of course, by definition, but its presence does not automatically mean that treatment is indicated. If the patient has symptoms and there is documented growth in the amount of fluid, then it pushes us towards treatment, but likewise, an asymptomatic patient with a slip of SRF that seems stable and unchanging, or at least minimally changing, can indeed be monitored instead. It alone is much less damaging to the retina, and an argument can be made that anti-VEGF injections could potentially do more harm than leaving it.

Finally, sub-RPE fluid such as PEDs are the lowest-risk lesions of all. In fact, an RPE detachment is not grounds for treatment alone, though the presence of features such a prechoroidal cleft may indeed mean that the membrane is technically active.

Christiana Says...

Not all superheroes have capes. Similarly, not all SRF is secondary to a neovascular complex in AMD. It is important to highlight scenarios where there is the presence of SRF, often a sliver, but no neovascularisation. Recently, Hilely et al. described three patterns of non-neovascular fluid detected on spectral-domain OCT (SD-OCT) (3). First, a crest of fluid over the drusenoid PED; second, a pocket of fluid at the angle of a large druse or within the crypts of confluent drusen; and third, the draping of low-lying fluid over confluent drusen. This non-neovascular fluid pattern is hypothesised to be transudation rather than exudation. From clinical experience, these cases are not common, but they illustrate the need to demonstrate a neovascular lesion and assess and reassess for response to anti-VEGF therapy early in the treatment course in nAMD. If there is no response, stop and reassess.

DIAGNOSIS

Again, this mirrors the diagnosis of dry AMD because the very first tenet of that diagnosis is excluding wet AMD. To start with, a history the duration of visual loss, if present and noticed by the patient, tends to be much quicker and more devastating than with dry AMD. However, with non-neovascular disease, patients are more often than not unable to state a specific time period over which their vision has been deteriorating and state 'years' or 'a long time'. If conversion to wet AMD has occurred, patients often report things such as 'Tuesday three weeks ago', 'just before Christmas' or 'two months past'. Likewise, distortion is much more commonly noticed and patients report blinds, doors and windows or the edges of things being kicked out of shape. The acuity is of course important because if thinking about potential treatment, it is important to make sure the patient is still actually within range for anti-VEGF injections, the limit reimbursed in the UK being 1.20 LogMAR, though a moralistic grey area does exist a little to either side. There is no moral or medical barrier at the good end of the vision; having vision 'too good' to initiate treatment is an oxymoron and in this day and age rather than punishing the patient for presenting early by denying treatment until some arbitrary threshold has been passed, the correct response is to praise them for the care and attention that they pay their health.

OCT should always be performed with suspected nAMD with emphasis placed on noticing any of the features mentioned above, namely IRF, SRF, bleeding and RPE disruption or detachment. OCT-A, or increasingly rarely nowadays FFA, is then used to look for a membrane in the suspicious location. If everything else fits though, history and OCT findings, not finding an obvious CNVM membrane on OCT-A is not a game changer. Sometimes the membrane is not visible due to thickness of fluid, masking by blood, technological impediments or the skill of the photographer. An OCT-A assists you, but isn't the golden ticket.

Remember, FFAs are from the pre-OCT era, where the levels of detail you could see with the human eye alone is not really sufficient. FFAs nowadays should only be reserved for peculiar cases where the diagnosis is in doubt, such as possible cystoid macular oedema secondary to a uveitic process perhaps, or suspected PIC or other lesion with a secondary CNVM, or MNVM, to use a modern term. ICG is technically the only proper manner for diagnosing a type 3 CNVM due to the anastomosis between retinal and choroidal circulation being visible. However, because, in effect, it makes no real difference whether treatment is given or what treatment that might be, there is no real point in considering it here.

Artificial intelligence (AI) is an emerging technology that is said will eventually take over the interpretation of images, such that the role of the ophthalmologist will be relegated to perhaps reading the summary report in the same way we do with electrophysiology tests now. AI-based monitoring of neovascular AMD using fluid quantification in OCT has been incorporated into clinical practice in some clinics around the world, with commercialised options such as Retinsight. These systems are being used to accurately quantify IRF, SRF and PED from OCT scans, track response to anti-VEGF therapy over time, and may even be used to forecast disease progression and personalise therapy intervals (Schmidt-Erfurth et al. 2020). There are still barriers and challenges to introducing these tools in the National Health Service (NHS) largely due to the revenue model and intricacies around information governance. However, it would seem a matter of 'when' not 'if'. It must be remembered, though, that electrophysiology is still analysed by a qualified clinician and AI still has a way to go; whilst it is very good at run-of-the-mill scans, there is a disturbing tendency for when it goes wrong to go very wrong indeed. Plus, with many United Kingdom units finding even simple technology such as email and electronic patient records filled with bugs and various problems, don't hold your breath for the AI takeover happening any time soon.

Christiana Says...

PCV is a subtype of nAMD characterized by nodular dilatations arising from neovascular networks that ramify mainly in the subretinal pigment epithelial space and which are seen best on ICGA. It is essentially a variant of type 1 MNVM. The prevalence of PCV in Asia is estimated at approximately 50%, whilst this is 10–20% in White populations, although the latter may be underestimated due to infrequent use of ICGA. There appear to be differences in the phenotypes of PCV based on ethnicity, with the prevalence of drusen, pachychoroid disease and submacular haemorrhages differing by ethnicity. Delineating PCV as a subtype is important because intravitreal anti-VEGF therapy may control exudation from these lesions, but the effect on closure of the polypoidal structures can be variable and additional treatment with PDT may be required. It is therefore helpful to have a non-invasive rapid way of identifying these cases, and OCT, again, comes to the rescue. The features in

Figure 4.10 have a high sensitivity and specificity for detecting PCV on OCT; if still in doubt, proceed to ICGA. Table 4.1 illustrates the OCT features of PCV.

MANAGEMENT

Whilst in the past argon laser or PDT were considered viable treatments, these are almost never considered nowadays because they have been shown to be inadequate compared to intravitreal anti-VEGF agents. They can be safely dismissed as options for us coal face clinicians. The choice is twofold: (1) whether to treat and (2) which anti-VEGF agent to use if you and the patient think that treatment is the way forward. Whether to treat is a big decision. There is no cure for nAMD in the proper sense; a treat-and-extend course of anti-VEGF injections last for many years, sometimes the rest of the patient's life, and entails a lot of bother for the patient coming back and forth to the hospital, let alone enduring the injections themselves. In the same way that chronic obstructive pulmonary disease (COPD) has no cure and inhalers are taken for many

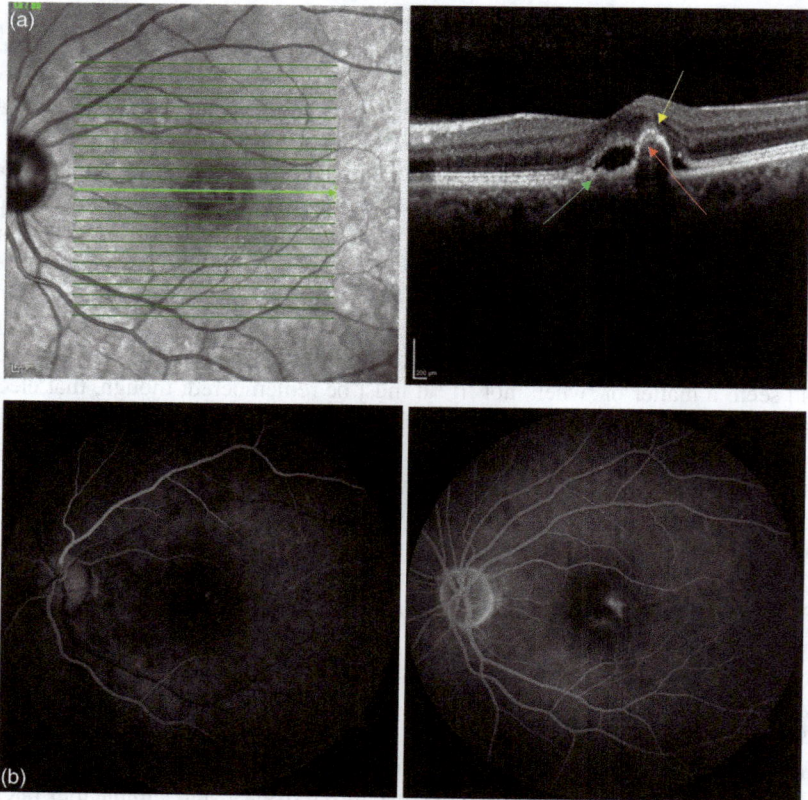

FIGURE 4.10   (a) Features of IPCV on OCT. Yellow arrow: Sharp-peaked (thumb-like PED). Red arrow: Hyperreflective lesion underlying the PED. Green arrow: double-layer sign. (b) IPCV on FFA. (c) Focal, nodular hyperfluorescence in the early and late phases with leakage on ICGA. *(Continued)*

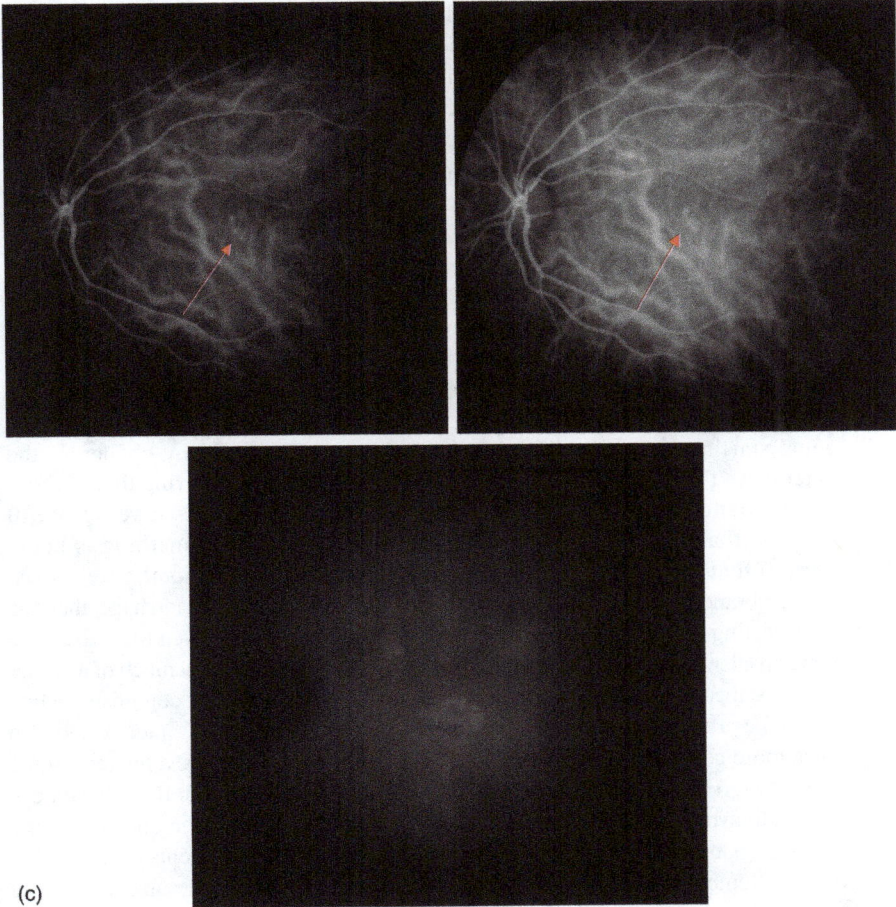

(c)

FIGURE 4.10 *(Continued)*

TABLE 4.1

Features Associated with OCT Diagnosis of PCV (4)

OCT Features of PCV – Major Criteria

Sub-RPE ring-like structure on cross-sectional OCT

Complex RPE elevation on en-face OCT

Sharp-peaked PED on cross-sectional OCT

Minor Criteria

Orange nodule

Thick choroid with dilated Haller's layer

Complex or multilobular PED

Double-layer sign

years if not forever, patients need to know that treatment is likely to be long-term. It is worth driving this point home as many patients still think, despite direct knowledge of the condition and the experience of increasing numbers of family and friends undergoing treatment, that there is still some distinct end point that will eventually be reached.

Pointing out the chronic nature of the condition and treatment is important when taking informed consent, and especially so in deciding whether to start treatment in borderline low-risk cases. Patients with low-grade type 1 CNVMs with only a slip of SRF and no IRF or haemorrhage might go years without worsening or even settle down spontaneously with no treatment. A judgement call can be made here depending on whether the patient is symptomatic, which would increase the chances of initiating treatment being in their best interest, and whether they are trustworthy and sensible with regard to monitoring, which would decrease the chance. Whilst nAMD most often progresses and causes permanent visual disability, this is not always the case, and the presence of a membrane associated with SRF alone does not automatically equal starting treatment. There are membranes discovered by chance in the contralateral eye that have no signs of activity and are just quietly sitting there. These are always monitored and never treated because injections would serve no useful purpose other than convincing the patient and the doctor that 'something is being done', even if that something is causing more potential harm than good.

If the membrane present is more aggressive and has IRF and/or haemorrhage, then the benefits of treating as opposed to monitoring vastly increase, though even then, there are important considerations. It is always important to take into account how much of a bother it would be for the patient to regularly attend as physical disabilities or cognitive decline might make the process of injection increasingly difficult for the patient, injector and also the service more generally. Always ask if treatment is in the patient's best interest. Some patients are so terrified of the process that they elect to let the vision in the affected eye be sacrificed to avoid the psychological burden of treatment. What is the point of having good vision if your whole life is spent worrying about upcoming treatments or recovering from the last. Sometimes general practitioners (GPs) prescribe anxiolytics and sometimes these are effective, but not always. So, on occasion, the kindest treatment is no treatment. If the vision is already impaired in the other eye and the eye affected is the only 'good' eye, the patient has the balance of judgement again because the consequences of not initiating prompt treatment are much more catastrophic. Even then, one of the authors remembers well a case of a patient undergoing monthly injections of an anti-VEGF agent for nAMD who took her own life rather than continue to endure treatment. Sometimes 'endure' is indeed the right word. Life is nuanced, and the right answer from a medical perspective is not always the right answer from a social perspective.

Once it is decided that intravitreal injection treatment is to be initiated, we then decide which regime to use and which drug. Regime-wise, there is only really one show in town; treat and extend. The alternatives are fixed dosing and pro re nata (PRN). With fixed dosing, as the name implies, injections are given at fixed intervals per the major studies, regardless of whether the macula is dry or not. This goes on forever with no end. The benefit is that this is simple to implement and run, but the downside is that it is resource heavy and patients end up overtreated, which is bad from both a patient experience and health economic perspective. So outside of clinical trials, fixed dosing regimes should be avoided. The PRN regime, by contrast, is very cost-efficient; patients are underdosed because injections are only administered if the OCT scan reveals activity. Therefore, the condition is allowed to deteriorate as a condition for treatment. The benefit is that money spent on drugs is saved, but the downside is that things are inefficient as more clinic visits are required, and the patients must come every 4 weeks or so forever and end up with worse vision. So, the only regime that should be used from an ethical, moral and cost-effective perspective during the initiation and maintenance phase is to treat and extend.

But what is treat and extend? As with fixed dosing, an injection is given at every visit with the key difference being that the intervals between injections are, as the name implies, extended or contracted in either 2- or 4-week aliquots depending on whether the eye is inactive or not. The benefits are that the clinics are easier to plan and cost-effective, but more importantly, that patients come as infrequently as possible for treatment while keeping the disease under control. It is the best of all worlds and should be the default regime everywhere. The below flowchart provides a scheme you can follow from diagnosis to management.

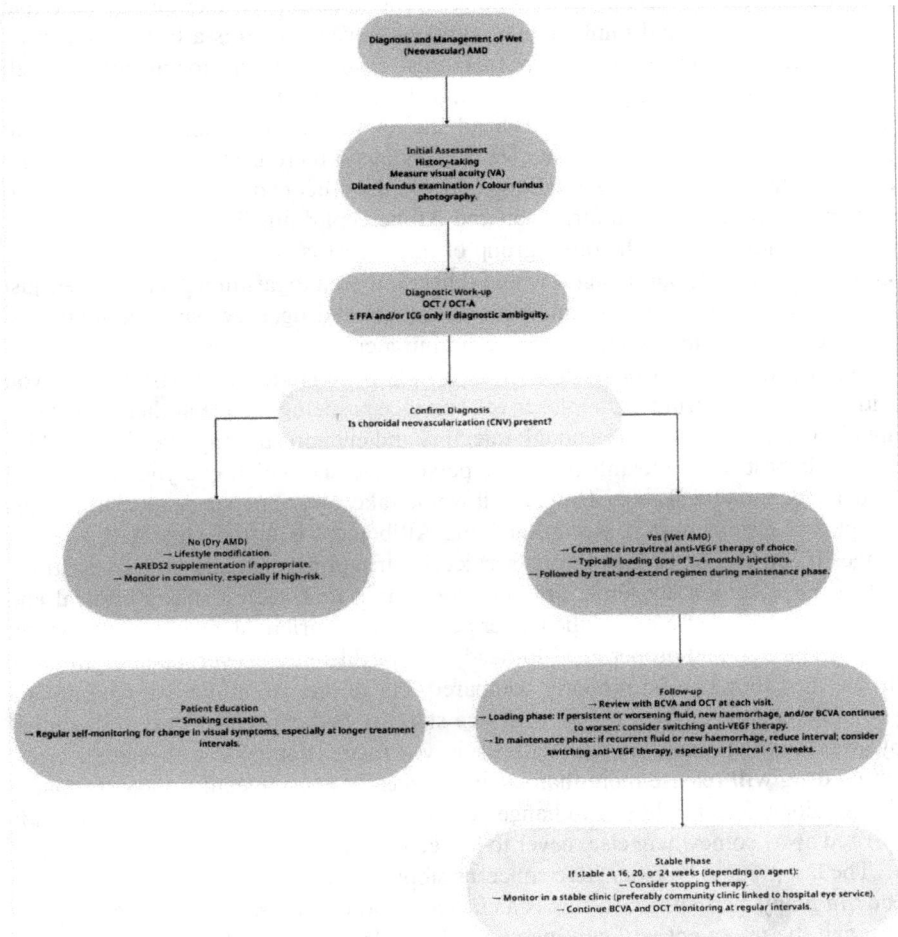

Diagnosis and Management of Wet (Neovascular) AMD

Initial Assessment
History-taking
Measure visual acuity (VA)
Dilated fundus examination / Colour fundus photography.

Diagnostic Work-up
OCT / OCT-A
± FFA and/or ICG only if diagnostic ambiguity.

Confirm Diagnosis
Is choroidal neovascularization (CNV) present?

No (Dry AMD)
— Lifestyle modification.
— AREDS2 supplementation if appropriate.
— Monitor in community, especially if high-risk.

Yes (Wet AMD)
— Commence intravitreal anti-VEGF therapy of choice.
— Typically loading dose of 3–4 monthly injections.
— Followed by treat-and-extend regimen during maintenance phase.

Patient Education
— Smoking cessation.
— Regular self-monitoring for change in visual symptoms, especially at longer treatment intervals.

Follow-up
— Review with BCVA and OCT at each visit.
— Loading phase: If persistent or worsening fluid, new haemorrhage, and/or BCVA continues to worsen; consider switching anti-VEGF therapy.
— In maintenance phase: if recurrent fluid or new haemorrhage, reduce interval; consider switching anti-VEGF therapy, especially if interval < 12 weeks.

Stable Phase
If stable at 16, 20, or 24 weeks (depending on agent):
— Consider stopping therapy.
— Monitor in a stable clinic (preferably community clinic linked to hospital eye service).
— Continue BCVA and OCT monitoring at regular intervals.

The final major choice to be made, and also the most controversial, is which drug to use. There are megabucks at stake here for big players, so it is difficult to find true head-to-head studies comparing things. Ideally, as clinicians, we should insist on true head-to-head, well-designed studies before we switch our practice from an established gold standard. In a nutshell, there is a sliding scale of drug choice available from ranibizumab 0.5% in 0.05 ml, either in the form of Lucentis or a biosimilar, to 2 mg aflibercept in 0.05 ml in the form of Eylea or a biosimilar; to more concentrated longer-acting agents such as 8 mg aflibercept (Eylea) in 0.07 ml and 6 mg faricimab (Vabysmo) in 0.05 ml There is also 1.25 mg bevacizumab (Avastin) in 0.05 ml, by far the nAMD staple throughout the world with the curious exception of the United Kingdom (long story) and 6 mg brolucizumab (Beovu), which has now fallen almost entirely out of favour because of concerns over high rates of adverse events such as blinding vasculitis.

There are two classes of drugs that can be used: cheaper biosimilars or longer-acting, more expensive agents. If you ask which of the cheaper ones is best, the answer is that in all probability, 2 mg of Aflibercept is the best, but there isn't really that much between that and ranibizumab, although bevacizumab is a little way behind again. The core difference is that bevacizumab tends not to dry the macular as well as ranibizumab, resulting in approximately 1 extra injection per year with bevacizumab as demonstrated in head-to-head studies funded by national institutes, but this saving comes at a significant cost (5). But again there isn't much in it. Nothing fundamental, despite what you will be told. On the other end of the scale, there is no known difference between faricimab and Aflibercept 8 mg. They are both stronger and longer lasting than the other group of three, that is certain, and by a clinically significant amount, but it isn't a whole other step on a logarithmic scale better, just better. Because they both have more molar amount of drug, they may be more immunogenic, resulting in potential increases in intraocular inflammation.

Academic types get bogged down in details from studies and will confuse you with stats, but the truth is simple. If your service is seeing people at their scheduled appointment time, you have enough injectors and enough capacity, then using a biosimilar is best from a health economic perspective and which one you choose will be dependent on local costs. However, it would take a lot to persuade most clinicians to opt for bevacizumab if biosimilar 2 mg Aflibercept is in the same ballpark cost range. If, on the other hand, your service is struggling, patients are not on time, delays are common and there are not enough injectors, then a strong clinical and moral case is made for one of the longer-acting drugs, faricimab or 8 mg Aflibercept. Once (if) a true and proper head-to-head, real-world study is ever made of all these drugs, then they can be properly compared, but in the meantime, we recommend you make a choice based on your service stability and capacity. Don't be beguiled by sweet-talking managers who will assure you that switching to a cheaper, shorter-acting drug will release more than enough funds for extra injectors and extra injection sessions. You might short-change your patients while the extra cash released is spirited away somewhere else, never to be seen again.

The last point to be made here concerns stopping treatment. When does treatment end? In many, perhaps most, this is a chronic condition present in the aged population and the treatment will continue unto death. In some, it will settle for a period, and in others, it will settle never to return again. Therefore, the algorithm you use must have a potential exit point. Whole life sentences were ruled very inadvisable in EU law. The most common regime is to have a loading phase of three (sometimes four) injections separated by 4 weeks, then if the macula is dry, extensions in the intervals can be made in 2- or 4-week steps up to 16 weeks (sometimes 20). Should the nAMD become active before reaching the magic 16-week (or 20) endpoint, then the interval can be reduced by 2 weeks until a sweet spot, if found, where the injections are given frequently enough to control the disease but infrequently enough that it causes the patient and service the least inconvenience. After a set number (there is no clear evidence) of injections at your chosen endpoint, a 'monitoring' phase can be entered where injections are withheld and OCTs are done at say 3-month intervals to catch any signs of reactivation, so the disease can be brought rapidly back under control. The exact means of arranging this has not been explored in a proper evidence-based manner on a regime-by-regime basis, so the honest truth is that it's up to you how you arrange it. However, when you put together an algorithm, make sure it's clear and everyone knows what it is.

Christiana Says...

Some key points before we delve into a summary of the main pivotal trials. The trials establishing intravitreal anti-VEGF therapy as the standard of treatment for nAMD were ANCHOR and MARINA (6,7). The eligibility criteria and the primary outcomes for these trials remain the benchmark for regulatory bodies and many payers in retinal trials. Knowledge of these factors also helps contextualise some of the real-world scenarios we see daily in clinic, and where later pragmatic trials and real-world evidence have helped and continue to help fill the gap.

The ANCHOR trial: Included eyes with predominantly classic subfoveal CNVM lesions, which were treated with ranibizumab or PDT. The baseline best corrected visual acuity (BCVA) had to be 6/12 or worse. The primary outcome was a proportion gaining 15 letters or more. In the ranibizumab arm, 40% gained 15 letters or more at 12 months, whereas only 6% gained 15 letters or more in the PDT arm.

The MARINA trial: Included eyes with minimally classic or occult CNVM lesions, which were treated with ranibizumab or sham injection. The baseline BCVA criteria and the primary outcome were the same as the ANCHOR trial. In the ranibizumab arm, 33.8% gained 15 letters or more, compared to 5% in the sham arm.

These two trials heralded the anti-VEGF era and have ushered in an age where we talk in terms of vision gained and not slowing of vision loss as we did pre-anti-VEGF therapy for nAMD. Table 4.2 illustrates the subsequent key trials associated with important drugs (8–11).

INJECTIONS SERVICES

How the service is arranged is key to success. An efficient injection system is sacrosanct, with enough capacity and enough non-medical practitioners to do the job comfortably. Following the doctrine of 'only do what only you can do', it really is an immoral case of economic sabotage for doctors to be undertaking injections in this day and age, and for actual consultants to be doing this is unconscionable. Doctors are few and far between and their time is valuable; far better to use non-medical practitioners,

TABLE 4.2

The Important Features of Key Trials Associated with anti-VEGF Agents

	View1 and View2	Hawk and Harrier	Tenaya and Lucerne	Pulsar
Intervention	Aflibercept 0.5 mg, 4 weekly Aflibercept 2 mg, 4 weekly Aflibercept 2 mg, 8 weekly (after 3 monthly doses)	Brolucizumab 3 mg Brolucizumab 6 mg Dosed monthly × 3, then treat and extend to 12-week intervals	Faricimab 6 mg after 4 monthly dosing – treat and extend to 16-week intervals	• Aflibercept 8 mg dosed monthly × 3 then extend to 12-week intervals. • Aflibercept 8 mg dosed monthly then extended to 16-week intervals. • Both arms could be shortened to 8-week intervals.
Comparator	Ranibizumab 0.5 mg 4 weekly	Aflibercept 2 mg Dosed monthly × 3 Then fixed dosing 8 weekly	Aflibercept 2 mg dosed monthly × 3, then fixed dosing 8 weekly	Eylea 2 mg dosed monthly ×3 then extended to 8 weeks fixed dosing
Mechanism of action of agent	Decoy receptor. Aflibercept competes with natural receptors VEGFR-1, VEGFR-2 to bind VEGF-A, VEGF-B and PIGF, preventing their actions on endothelial cells.	Single chain fragment of humanized monoclonal antibody – so much smaller than other agents. Binds with high affinity to all isoforms of VEGF-A		Same mechanism of action as Aflibercept – the quadruple dose is designed to increase durability.
No. of participants	2457	1817	1329	1009
Key eligibility criteria	1. Active subfoveal CNVM secondary to AMD 2. Visual acuity between 6/96 and 6/12 3. Treatment –naïve eyes only	Similar to VIEW1 and VIEW 2 but visual acuity criteria was up to 78 ETDRS letters (approximately 6/7.5).	Similar to VIEW1 and VIEW2 but visual acuity eligibility up to 78 ETDRS letters (6/7.5)	Similar to VIEW1 and VIEW2 Visual acuity eligibility up to 78 letters

(Continued)

TABLE 4.2 *(Continued)*
The Important Features of Key Trials Associated with anti-VEGF Agents

	View1 and View2	Hawk and Harrier	Tenaya and Lucerne	Pulsar
Primary Outcome	95–96% maintained vision at week 52 defined as proportion losing <15 ETDRS letters from baseline	Mean BCVA change at week 48 was +6.6 ; +6.9 (brolucizumab 6 mg), + 6.1 (brolucizumab 3 mg) vs +6.8; +7.6 (Aflibercept)	Mean BCVA change at week 40–48 average: +5.8; +6.6 (faricimab), +5.1; +6.6 (Aflibercept)	Mean BCVA change at week 48 Aflibercept 2 mg: +7.6 Aflibercept 8 mg at 12 weeks: +6.7 Aflibercept 8 mg at 16 weeks: +6.2
Importance and practice implications	Demonstrated equivalence to ranibizumab, with the 8-week regimen sustaining efficacy offering a significant reduction in treatment burden	Brolucizumab demonstrated non-inferiority to Aflibercept. Brolucizumab demonstrated sustained drying compared to Aflibercept, but up to 5% intraocular inflammation compared to 1% with Aflibercept.	Faricimab demonstrated non-inferiority to Aflibercept. Efficacy was maintained in the faricimab arm with extended dosing. Note the Aflibercept arm was not similarly extended.	Aflibercept 8 mg demonstrated non-inferior visual gains compared to Aflibercept 2 mg every 8 weeks. Aflibercept 2 mg was not tested at 12- or 16-week intervals

usually employed at the band 6 level, to perform injections usually at a frequency of 16 per booked session. These should be undertaken in a proper clean room as opposed to an operating theatre, which can then be released for more appropriate procedures such as cataract surgery. There should be enough redundancy in the system that injectors are not overworked and that everyone is seen at their appointment time, which is essential in a treat-and-extend regime. If there is slippage in appointments, then the whole system becomes utterly meaningless and even worse than PRN.

Whichever drug is chosen, there is little sense in having many drugs used simultaneously. This will lead to confusion and an increased likelihood of the wrong drug being injected. Standardisation of rules, regime and drug leads to success. Having different consultants in the department doing things slightly differently for ego's sake or simple bloody-mindedness is a recipe for disaster. Standardise, standardise, standardise! Consultants should be approachable and available to answer questions and queries that come up, and there will always be issues; otherwise, confusion leads to paralysis and paralysis leads to mistakes. The role of a consultant should therefore be that of a benign overseer, wandering around the clinic like the Victorian factory managers of old, keeping a close eye on things and being seen to do so.

Audits are important in maintaining standards of excellence. Always checking patients are satisfied, visual results are good, referral to treatment times are 2 weeks or fewer, complication rates are acceptable and patients are seen at their appointment times. Non-medical practitioners can be used to see follow-up patients and perform yearly review clinics, checking pressures and cataracts and generally check on how things are doing; this will then release doctors to do other things, though far more commonly, there would not have been enough doctors to do these tasks in the first place.

Christiana Says...

Whilst the anti-VEGF era has been transformational, reducing irreversible sight loss due to nAMD reduced by 30–50% in most regions, the results attained in real-world clinic settings trail behind the trials. There are many important contributory factors to this, including the significant heterogeneity of treatment response and treatment needs across patient populations. Another key factor is the significant infrastructure required to deliver these treatments as described in the pivotal studies. Over the years, clinicians have evolved treatment regimens to maximise clinical efficacy within the constraints of health services. It was evident from the pivotal trials that the maximal visual acuity gain occurs after the first 3 monthly injections, therefore the natural evolution was to introduce a loading dose of 3 monthly injections and monthly review with treatment at reactivation. This was first reported in the Prospective Optical Coherence Tomography Imaging of patients with neovascular AMD Treated with Intraocular ranibizumab (PrONTO study). Table 4.3 illustrates different treatment regimes used in different studies.

The PrONTO study pioneered the idea of individualized treatment regimens, moving away from fixed monthly injections. However, in real-world settings, PRN dosing often lead to fewer injections than ideal, fluctuations in retinal exudation and cumulative damage over time. Many studies (such as CATT and IVAN) showed better outcomes with regular/frequent dosing than PRN. This highlights the difficulties in translating

TABLE 4.3
Differing Treatment Regimes in Different Studies

	Fixed Dosing	PRN Regime	Loading + Quarterly Loading	Treat and Extend
Landmark trial	ANCHOR and MARINA	PRONTO study (12)	PIER study (13)	LUCAS TREX-AMD (14,15)
Dosing regime	Fixed monthly dosing	Monthly loading for 3 months and then PRN	Monthly loading for 3 months and then quarterly fixed dosing	TREX-AMD: Monthly ranibizumab 0.5 mg until dry macula achieved followed by 2-week extensions to max of 12 weeks vs monthly ranibizumab LUCAS: Ranibizumab 0.5 mg vs Avastin 1.25 mg. Both arms on a treat-and-extend basis

clinical trials into real-world practice, with participants in the PrONTO study reviewed monthly, OCTs at every monthly visit, and highly trained staff, and a reading centre monitoring closely. This is difficult or impossible to replicate in the real world.

Treat and extend emerged as a proactive treatment regime that reduces the monitoring burden and customises the treatment interval and remains the most commonly used treatment regime presently. Studies like TREX-AMD, LUCAS and ALTAIR showed that treat and extend is non-inferior to monthly dosing in maintaining visual gains.

Other authors have explored the use of OCT biomarkers to identify predictors of response, especially in the context of large variability in response and treatment requirement. Whilst many such biomarkers have been explored, a recent meta-analysis evaluating more than 80 distinct OCT biomarkers determined that the presence of an intact external limiting membrane and intact ellipsoid zone predicted better visual acuity at 12 months. Easy to remember. In contrast, the presence of baseline IRF at the foveal centre point and the presence of subretinal hyperreflective material, GA, and PED predicted worse visual acuity at 12 months (16).

It is not the purview of this book to go into detail about therapies that are as yet unlicensed and may never be, but Table 4.4 illustrates current studies and the drugs

TABLE 4.4
Promising Therapies in Phase 3 Trial for nAMD

Therapy	Mechanism of Action	Frequency of Administration	Pivotal Trial
Duravyu (Vorolanib implant)	Tyrosine kinase inhibitor. It functions by inhibiting all VEGF receptors. It also inhibits the platelet-derived growth factor receptor (PDGFR).	6 monthly by intravitreal injection	Lugano & Lucia
Axpaxli (Axitinib)	Tyrosine kinase inhibitor. Inhibits all VEGF receptors and PDGFR	6 monthly by intravitreal injection	SOL1 and SOL-R
RGX-314	Gene therapy. It uses a recombinant adeno-associated virus vector to deliver the gene encoding an anti-VEGF fragment.	Once by subretinal injection requiring vitrectomy or suprachoroidal injection in clinic	ASCENT
Susvimo (Port delivery system, ranibizumab)	This surgical implant contains a reservoir that continuously releases ranibizumab at a controlled rate.	Surgical implant with 6–9 monthly refill	ARCHWAY
4D-150	It uses an adeno-associated virus vector engineered to deliver the gene expressing Aflibercept and to interfere and block VEGF-C.	Once by intravitreal injection	4FRONT 1 & 2

they are testing so that you can undertake further reading if needed, or in case you want to impress a colleague by dropping in the name of a drug they almost certainly know nothing about.

It is an exciting time indeed in the world of nAMD, illustrating nicely the enduring scientific, clinical and intellectual challenge that is the world of medical retina!

REFERENCES

1. De Oliveira Dias JR et al. Natural history of subclinical neovascularisation in non-exudative age-related macular degeneration using swept-source OCT angiography. Ophthalmology. 2018; 125:255–266.
2. Sacconi R et al. Towards a better understanding of non-exudative choroidal and macular neovascularisation. Prog Retin Eye Res. 2023; 92:101113.
3. Hilely A et al. Non-neovascular age-related macular degeneration with subretinal fluid. Br J Ophthalmol. 2021; 105(10):1415–1420.
4. Cheung CMG, Lai TYY, Teo K, Ruamviboonsuk P, Chen SJ, Kim JE, Gomi F, Koh AH, Kokame G, Jordan-Yu JM, Corvi F, Invernizzi A, Ogura Y, Tan C, Mitchell P, Gupta V, Chhablani J, Chakravarthy U, Sadda SR, Wong TY, Staurenghi G, Lee WK. Polypoidal choroidal vasculopathy: Consensus nomenclature and non-indocyanine green angiograph diagnostic criteria from the Asia-Pacific Ocular imaging society PCV workgroup. Ophthalmology. 2021; 128(3):443–452. doi: 10.1016/j.ophtha.2020.08.006. Epub 2020 Aug 11.
5. Martin DF, Maguire MG, Fine SL, Ying G-S, Jaffe GJ, Grunwald JE, Toth C, Ferris FL; CATT Research Group. Ranibizumab and bevacizumab for treatment of neovascular age-related macular degeneration: Two-year results. Ophthalmology. 2012; 119(7):1388–1398.
6. Rosenfeld PJ, Brown DM, Heier JS, Boyer DS, Kaiser PK, Chung CY, Kim RY; MARINA Study Group. Ranibizumab for neovascular age-related macular degeneration. N Engl J Med. 2006; 355(14):1419–1431. doi: 10.1056/NEJMoa054481.
7. Brown DM, Michels M, Kaiser PK, Heier JS, Sy JP, Ianchulev T. Ranibizumab versus verteporfin photodynamic therapy for neovascular age-related macular degeneration: Two-year results of the ANCHOR study. Ophthalmology. 2009; 116:57–65.e5.
8. Lanzetta P, Korobelnik JF, Heier JS, Leal S, Holz FG, Clark WL, Eichenbaum D, Iida T, Xiaodong S, Berliner AJ, Schulze A, Schmelter T, Schmidt-Ott U, Zhang X, Vitti R, Chu KW, Reed K, Rao R, Bhore R, Cheng Y, Sun W, Hirshberg B, Yancopoulos GD, Wong TY; PULSAR Investigators. Intravitreal aflibercept 8 mg in neovascular age-related macular degeneration (PULSAR): 48-week results from a randomised, double-masked, non-inferiority, phase 3 trial. Lancet. 2024; 403(10432):1141–1152. doi: 10.1016/S0140-6736(24)00063-1. Epub 2024 Mar 7.
9. Heier JS, Khanani AM, Quezada Ruiz C, Basu K, Ferrone PJ, Brittain C, Figueroa MS, Lin H, Holz FG, Patel V, Lai TYY, Silverman D, Regillo C, Swaminathan B, Viola F, Cheung CMG, Wong TY; TENAYA and LUCERNE Investigators. Efficacy, durability, and safety of intravitreal faricimab up to every 16 weeks for neovascular age-related macular degeneration (TENAYA and LUCERNE): Two randomised, double-masked, phase 3, non-inferiority trials. Lancet. 2022; 399(10326):729–740. doi: 10.1016/S0140-6736(22)00010-1. Epub 2022 Jan 24.
10. Dugel PU, Koh A, Ogura Y, Jaffe GJ, Schmidt-Erfurth U, Brown DM, Gomes AV, Warburton J, Weichselberger A, Holz FG; HAWK and HARRIER Study Investigators. HAWK and HARRIER: Phase 3, multicenter, randomized, double-masked trials of brolucizumab for neovascular age-related macular degeneration. Ophthalmology. 2020; 127(1):72–84. doi: 10.1016/j.ophtha.2019.04.017. Epub 2019 Apr 12.

11. Heier JS, Brown DM, Chong V, Korobelnik JF, Kaiser PK, Nguyen QD, Kirchhof B, Ho A, Ogura Y, Yancopoulos GD, Stahl N, Vitti R, Berliner AJ, Soo Y, Anderesi M, Groetzbach G, Sommerauer B, Sandbrink R, Simader C, Schmidt-Erfurth U; VIEW 1 and VIEW 2 Study Groups. Intravitreal aflibercept (VEGF trap-eye) in wet age-related macular degeneration. Ophthalmology. 2012; 119(12):2537–2548. doi: 10.1016/j.ophtha.2012.09.006. Epub 2012 Oct 17. Erratum in: Ophthalmology. 2013 Jan;120(1):209-10.
12. Fung AE et al. An optical coherence tomography-guided, variable-dosing regimen with intravitreal ranibizumab (Lucentis) for neovascular age-related macular degeneration. Am J Ophthalmol. 2007; 143:566–583.
13. Regillo CD et al. Randomised, double-masked, sham-controlled trial of ranibizumab for neovascular age-related macular degeneration: PIER Study Year 1. Am J Ophthalmol. 2008; 145:239–248.
14. Berg K et al. Ranibizumab or bevacizumab for neovascular age-related macular degeneration according to the Lucentis Compared to Avastin Study treat and extend protocol: Two year results. Ophthalmology. 2016; 123(1):51–9.
15. Kertes PJ et al. Efficacy of a treat and extend regimen with Ranibizumab in patients with neovascular age-related macular disease: A randomised clinical trial. JAMA Ophthalmology. 2019; 138(3):314–321.
16. Nanji K et al. Baseline OCT biomarkers predicting visual outcomes in neovascular age-related macular degeneration: A meta-analysis. Ophthalmology. 2025; 132(11):1241–1252.
17. Ursula Schmidt-Erfurth et al. Application of automated quantification of fluid volumes to anti-VEGF therapy of neovascular age-related macular degeneration. Ophthalmology. 2020; 127(9):1211–1219

5 Myopic and Other Secondary Neovascular Membranes

As mentioned in Chapter 4, not all macular neovascular membranes (MNVMs) will be due to age-related macular degeneration (AMD). Fair enough; the majority are, and the treatment from the perspective of the membrane is the same, but there are important other considerations as well. If a patient is younger than most neovascular AMD (nAMD) patients, the question should always be asked, could this be due to something else? Of the so-called secondary choroidal neovascular membranes (CNVMs), or MNVMs, depending on which shibboleth you prefer, myopia is the most common cause. Others include pretty much anything that damages the RPE or Bruch's membrane complex – uveitis, trauma, genetic conditions, you name it. Anything that cracks the patio surface can result in a weed growing through the crack –weak patio tiles, excessive weight placed on it over time, a sharp knock from a collapsing barbecue or excessive weather. However, in reality, the difference between any of these causes and simple wear and tear of normal patio tiles that have aged over time is more of academic interest than anything else when it comes to treatment, but *not* when it comes to systemic implications and prognosis.

MYOPIC FUNDI

Myopic eyes are longer than usual, which is why they're myopic of course, and as the limited retinal pigment epithelium (RPE) and Bruch's membrane are stretched over a bigger and bigger area they're more likely to break in places that are termed 'lacquer cracks'. Lacquer is the term for a sort of glossy varnish that is applied when wet, but as it dries, it can crack as the material shrinks. They look like whitish lines in highly myopic fundi, more common around the disc and radiating from it, and provide opportunities for neovascular membranes to grow through into the retina. Figure 5.1 illustrates the appearance of lacquer cracks in a myopic fundus.

Myopic fundi generally look increasingly abnormal depending on the degree of myopia present. High myopia is classed as an eye with a refraction of greater than -6.00 diopters and in the mildest form, the fundus might have some peripapillary atrophy as the RPE struggles to stretch to the disc, with an increasingly tessellated fundus indicating increasing myopia. Tessellated is a word bandied around a lot, but nobody stops to explain what it is. Tessellation is another word for a mosaic-like appearance, where irregular tiles fit together to form a pattern on a wall with an even space between these little tiles and no overlap. This appearance is caused by the thinness of the RPE causing the choroidal vessels to be seen through the retina, breaking

DOI: 10.1201/9781003628309-5

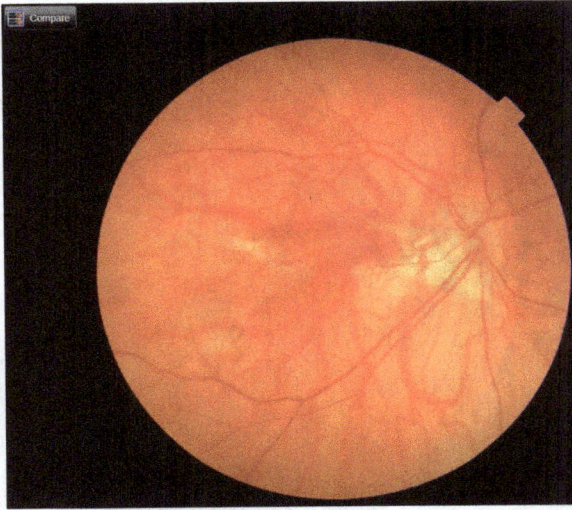

FIGURE 5.1   Lacquer cracks.

up the fundus into discrete little islands between these vessels. Normally, of course, the choroidal vessels cannot be seen. Perhaps a better term for the same phenomenon is 'tigroid' fundus, as in 'tiger-like', because the stripes formed by the choroidal vessels do look like a tiger's coat in a way. Perhaps this can be best remembered as a tessellated pattern of a tiger. Figure 5.2 illustrates a tessellated, or tigroid, fundus.

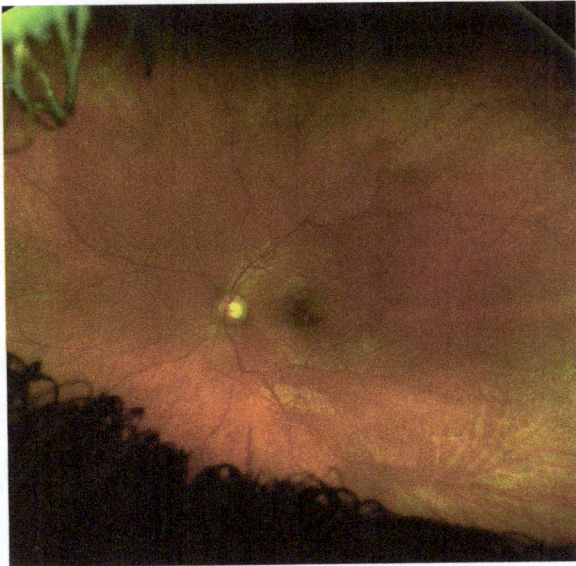

FIGURE 5.2   A tessellated, or tigroid, fundus.

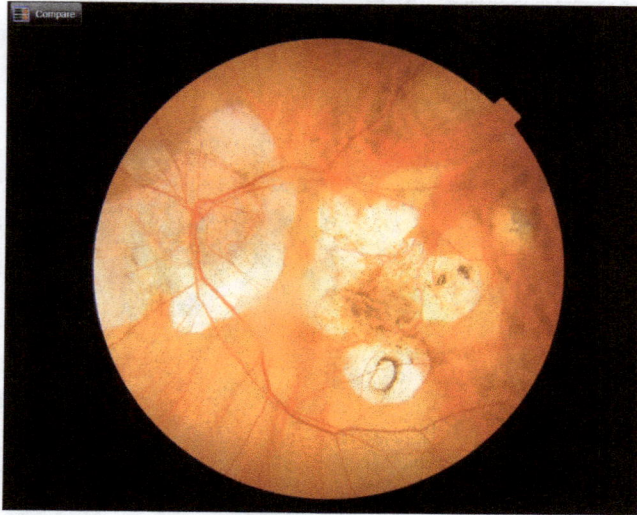

FIGURE 5.3   A myopic eye with chorioretinal atrophy.

As the degree of myopia increases, chorioretinal atrophy begins to appear, and as the name suggests, the choroid and retina both start thinning until eventually patches of white posterior sclera become starkly visible. There is a sliding scale of severity here from diffuse small dots in multiple areas to patchy bits of white to large slabs of white extending over much of the fundus, including the macula, with lines of remaining normal tissue separating the large white areas. Figure 5.3 illustrates an eye with extensive chorioretinal atrophy. Increasingly myopic eyes are more prone to posterior staphyloma development, with more than one properly called staphylomata, which is an out-pouching of the usually circular coat of the eye due to overstretching related weakness and thus peculiar anatomy. A form of posterior staphyloma that can occur in myopic eyes is called 'dome maculopathy'. In dome maculopathy, there is a dome-like submacular in-pouching of the wall of the eye, which can result in a slip of structural subretinal fluid appearing on the peak of the dome that all the anti–vascular endothelial growth factor (anti-VEGF) injections in all the world won't be able to shift (see below).

A stretched myopic eyeball can also result in what's called myopic foveoschisis, maculoschisis, or indeed any variant of this name, which simply means a splitting of the layers of the retina due to overstretching resulting in a distinctly structural-looking band of intraretinal fluid. Figure 5.4 demonstrates a macula with myopic schitic appearance. The primary importance of knowing about this isn't to know how to treat it but to know that it isn't caused by exudation or by CNVM, so again, as with dome maculopathy, avoid useless injections at all costs; they won't make a difference here. (It's very difficult to treat this condition, though some regard some complex forms of vitreoretinal surgery as the answer; but unless you hate your vitreoretinal colleagues, don't refer the patient to them for treatment.) Other forms of degenerative scarring, or gliosis, can occur too, such as epiretinal membrane formation and all

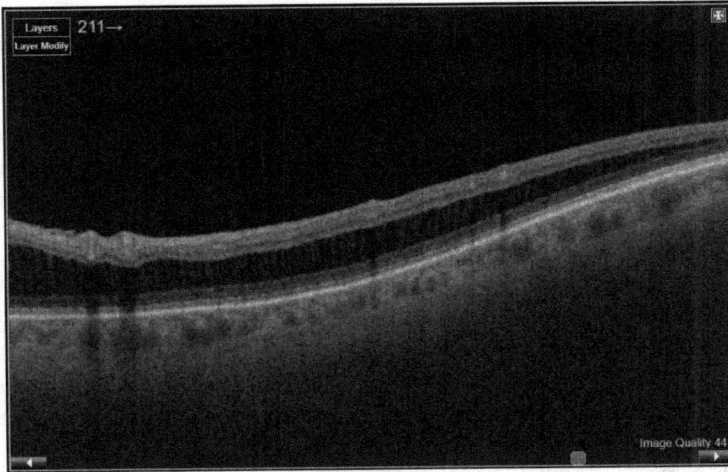

FIGURE 5.4   An optical coherence tomography (OCT) of a macula with myopic foveoschisis.

sorts of weird and wonderful vitreoretinal things, without even beginning to consider retinal tears, detachments and such.

The last thing to mention in this section, before going on to discuss the MNVM itself, is the Forster–Fuchs spot. This is a myopic variant of a disciform macular scar where, as a response to a haemorrhage caused by myopic CNVM, the RPE hypertrophies and a raised scar develops with a pigmented hue. This is a sign that there was activity in the past, but that activity has led to scarring.

Myopic fundi are indeed a minefield. The worrying thing is that worldwide trends indicate a rapidly increasing prevalence of myopia, including high myopia, among the young. There are many theories as to why this might be; close work, lack of playing outdoors, phone and iPad usage and exposure to the 'wrong' sort of ultraviolet light due to artificial bulbs giving off a spectrum of UV waves different from the sun, the bringer of all life. Obviously, the eye stops growing in childhood, so unless you work in paediatric ophthalmology, this might seem of academic interest alone. However, ultimately, it is a microcosm of other and all forms of ill health brought on by increasingly artificial living and our divorce from the natural world.

The current myopia epidemic will have an impact on retinal practice because we can expect to see more myopic CNVMs over time if the trend continues unabated.

MYOPIC NEOVASCULAR MEMBRANES

The neovascular membranes that occur in myopia are usually noticed far more readily by patients than those developing due to nAMD. This may be due to the fact that the patient cohort tends to be considerably younger, or it might be because of the disproportionate effect of fluid at a myopic macula, but whatever the reason, patients tend to be much more aware of distortion and blur, oftentimes much more so than the optical coherence tomography (OCT) scan might suggest. Sometimes patients complain bitterly of symptoms and the degree of macular abnormality is so mild that it confuses clinicians, who list the patient for cataract surgery, diagnose a posterior vitreous detachment or send them for exotic tests when a few weeks down the line it becomes clearer that a CNVM is developing.

OCT scans are generally a lot less striking than those with nAMD, though the myopic fundus will confuse things a bit as everything looks a bit strange with very thin choroid and the scan might be at a 45-degree angle or difficult to properly take and so blurry and affected by artefacts. Because the RPE and Bruch's membrane are both stretched and thin, the membranes that do form tend to be type 2 more than type 1, and the complex tends to be subretinal and present with an initial 'fluffy border'. This looks totally different from the very clear and symmetric border that an adult vitelliform lesion may form, though confusion can occur, but the typical fluffy border is, as described, fluffy, as in indistinct and difficult to delineate. OCT angiography (OCT-A) tends to show a clear membrane, which may be quite small, mainly because the condition tends to be caught relatively early.

Pitfalls here include not differentiating between a true myopic CNVM and benign structural conditions such as dome maculopathy or myopic foveoschisis. These are not exudative conditions at all and as such do not benefit one bit from injections. In myopic patients, be aware of these imposters and be humble. If a patient does not seem to derive any benefit from your course of injections, lovingly administered with care and well-meaning attention, you may be wrong about it being a true CNVM and must have the courage to suspend treatment to see what happens. If suspending treatment has as little effect on the fluid as starting it did, then chances are you're looking at a structural issue, not an exudative one.

Regarding prognosis, myopic membranes tend to be quite forgiving, with the proportion that settle down spontaneously without treatment being considerably higher than with nAMD. That said, treatment is of course best offered and offered early to avoid as much damage as possible to vision. While it is recognised that myopic membranes tend to settle quickly and are relatively forgiving, we would not suggest that you treat them any differently than regular membranes. At the end of the day, how can you know if a neovascular membrane is due to myopia, old age, or some combination of both? Myopic people get old, and older people can be myopic. So the added amount of danger and confusion that would result from trying to deduce whether a membrane is mainly due to myopia or not is simply not worth it. It is academic. Treat it the same as you would nAMD; with a treat and extend regime of anti-VEGF exactly as you would in the previous chapter. Never needlessly overcomplicate things.

The only special consideration that should be borne in mind, not just with myopic CNVM but with all secondary CNVMs and to a lesser extent nAMD as well, is that the younger patient age group presenting may include to a woman of potentially childbearing age being in need of a course of intravitreal anti-VEGF treatment. There is a lot of hysteria about the potential dangers of initiating or continuing intravitreal anti-VEGF treatment in a pregnant woman. Although the reality is that there is no real-world evidence that there is any danger, it is always best to check and to warn patients, both verbally and diligently recorded in the notes, of the potential dangers of any treatment to unborn children. The potential risks associated with

TABLE 5.1

The Two Landmark Trials for Therapeutic Agents in Myopic CNVM (1,2)

Trial Name	Trial Design	Outcome
RADIANT	12-month randomized, double-masked multicentre trial comparing intravitreal ranibizumab 0.5 mg 1 + PRN or 3 + PRN with photodynamic therapy (PDT) (could be switched to ranibizumab from month 3)	+13.8 – 14.4 vs +9.3 for PDT
MYRROR	Aflibercept 2 mg 1 + prn vs sham	+12.1 letter vs –2.0 in sham group at 24 weeks

anti-VEGF in pregnancy include potential impact on the placental vascular network and foetal development. In principle, ranibizumab has the shortest systemic half-life and clearance of the current anti-VEGF therapies and would be considered lower risk. Management in partnership with an obstetrician is advised.

Christiana Says...

Another potential differential for the uninitiated is a macular hole secondary to myopia, which can present with a cuff of intraretinal fluid on OCT. Importantly, this will not be associated with a hyperreflective lesion in the subretinal space, as you would see in actual myopic CNVM.

The natural history of myopic CNVM can result in macular atrophy and fibrosis, leading to irreversible visual loss in most eyes by 5 years. Long-term studies report visual acuity <1.00LogMAR in over 85% of untreated eyes by 5 years.

As you will see from the following, we have two agents with good results from well-designed randomized controlled trials (RCTs), so either can be used. There is no head-to-head comparison of these agents, so whichever is funded by your payer will do.

Table 5.1 summarises the two landmark trials for therapeutic agents in myopic CNVM.

The study design, which in both trials only mandates at least one intravitreal injection followed by a PRN regime, highlights the difference between myopic CNVM and the other vascular retinal diseases we have discussed thus far. This may be because in myopic CNVM, VEGF is upregulated acutely due to mechanical stresses rather than the chronic and sustained oxidative stress we see in nAMD.

SECONDARY MEMBRANES AS A RESULT OF UVEITIS

Uveitis is a broad church and contains a spectrum of inflammatory and infectious conditions that can damage the uveal tract. Anything that causes breaks or weaknesses in the RPE or Bruch's membrane cracks the patio, and weeds can then grow through that crack. The list is therefore legion and cannot possibly be described in its entirety here, or indeed anywhere. Notable causes include punctate inner choroidopathy (PIC), a condition of young usually myopic females that involves scarring at the macula in one, or even both eyes (Practical Uveitis: Understanding the Grape eBook: Williams, Gwyn Samuel, Westcott, Mark: Amazon.co.uk: Books).

Other conditions include multifocal choroiditis lesions, tuberculosis scars, serpiginous choroiditis lesions, acute posterior multifocal placoid pigment epitheliopathy and chorioretinal sarcoidosis scars. Any scarring process that leaves a weak spot through which CNVM can grow.

It is imperative to treat the uveitic condition itself, of course, but if a secondary CNVM has occurred, then it is important to recognise this for what it is rather than assume it must naturally be due to the effects of the inflammation. If the location of the lesion threatens the macula and therefore vision, then treatment may need to be instituted, though if the scar causing membrane growth is far enough away, then it might be possible to closely monitor things instead. All membranes eventually scar up and close in the same way that all bleeding eventually ends, but the important thing is to ensure key structures are protected. Sometimes a peripheral CNVM can occur secondary to age as well and as with all such peripheral lesions, these are much less readily noticed by the patient and ophthalmologist than anything around the macula. The term used to describe such lesions, particularly when they scar up, is 'eccentric disciform' because they are in an unusual location (therefore eccentric) and roundish in shape (therefore disciform).

Sudden changes in symptoms that are associated with new haemorrhage, intra-retinal, or subretinal fluid on OCT, in the presence of a pigmented retinal scar, must be assumed to be due to a secondary CNVM until proven otherwise. As with any neovascular membrane, timely treatment is key, and again the algorithm used should be no different from that used in all other membranes. Having separate algorithms and treatment plans for membranes derived from different conditions is a recipe for confusion and subsequent mistakes. Stick to the same plan; a neovascular membrane is a neovascular membrane.

PERIPAPILLARY CHOROIDAL NEOVASCULAR MEMBRANES

It is not hugely unusual to find small areas of fluid and/or blood around the optic nerve head during routine examination or while looking for something else when examining the eye. In fact, with so many optometrists looking into so many eyes so much of the time, it is really no wonder that all sorts of things are being discovered that previously lingered quietly in the back of the eye not causing any trouble to anyone. Naevi are the main discoveries, but we will discuss them in Chapter 10. Peripapillary choroidal neovascular membranes (PPCNVMs) is another. As the name suggests, these are neovascular membranes, but instead of being located at the macula, they are, as the name suggests, next to the optic disc. Most times, PPCNVMs do not cause symptoms; they are most often discovered by chance by an eagle-eyed optometrist determined to earn their silver by proving to the patient and possibly themselves that they have skills over and above any previous optometrist who may have seen the patient. Occasionally, patients report to primary or secondary care because they have noticed exactly the same constellation of symptoms that are experienced in nAMD, and are usually of the same age and risk factor group as regular macular degeneration patients, but mostly they are asymptomatic.

Examination of the disc might reveal fluid and/or small spots of blood around one of the margins, though in symptomatic patients, it might be the case that the fluid and blood is more extensive and stretch from the disc all the way to the fovea.

The OCT is surprisingly similar to that seen with nAMD, with RPE disruption and potential subretinal or intraretinal fluid present. OCT-A might reveal a type 1 or type 2 membrane, though polypoidal choroidal vasculopathy (PCV) might also rarely be the cause. The main and only thing to determine here is whether the membrane is threatening the fovea or not and whether it is symptomatic. Knowing that the membrane is usually derived not from a break in the RPE–Bruch complex as such, but degeneration that can occur as a specific result of how the RPE abuts the disc with a predilection for atrophy in this specific place, and hence the frequency relative to any other random extrafoveal location, is academic. In a nutshell, if the patient is symptomatic and the membrane is threatening the fovea, then treatment may be necessary, but if not, then monitoring may well be the answer. It really is as simple as that, with treatment if needed being exactly the same as that instituted for nAMD and myopic CNVM.

A good case might be made that any optometrist or indeed ophthalmologist finding an asymptomatic PPCNVM could give home monitoring advice and an Amsler grid and see on symptom. Sometimes the position of the fluid edge might be, say, halfway between the disc and fovea, and you might feel happier repeating the scan in 3 months or so to see if it's moved or not before discharging. If the membrane is on the nasal side, then obviously the risk is going to be as low as it gets. In view of the fact that only a small number of patients with PPCNVM need treatment and NHS clinics are usually overbooked and lacking capacity, it is not in anyone's best interest to follow these patients much longer than this. As many optometrists now have access to OCT, monitoring in the community is suitable here and it is preferred to monitoring by Amsler due to its low sensitivity. The risk of a sudden, sight-threatening subretinal or submacular haemorrhage is low with PPCNVM; however, it is not nil. A not-so-rare differential to consider when there is fluid adjacent to the optic nerve is peripapillary pachychoroid syndrome, which is a subtype within pachychoroid disease spectrum, with thickening of the choroid in the peripapillary region that may be associated with intraretinal fluid.

CHOROIDAL OSTEOMA

This is a peculiar condition where calcific bone-like material replaces the normal choroid in the eye of a teenager or young adult and is considered a benign tumour. It usually occurs in the peripapillary area of one eye but can extend to the macula on occasion. The overlying retina is, of course, denied its rightful blood supply and withers as a consequence, with profound impact on vision. Whilst some patients may be asymptomatic, most report gradually worsening blurring of vision with metamorphopsia, with this being very profound indeed if the macula is involved. Examination reveals a whitish or yellowish, oddly shaped plaque close to the disc that can be of any shape and extend in any direction. Nobody really knows why it happens because most occur in normal eyes, though it is hypothesised that inflammation, trauma or some kind of insult can set it off.

The gold standard diagnostic tool is B-scan ultrasound, which shows a bright signal, as would be expected of bone, right where the lesion is. Whilst other tests can reveal fascinating results, they are not useful and shouldn't really be used needlessly here if you think this is a choroidal osteoma, and it behaves exactly like it. There is no prevention and no treatment. Usually, because we are so unhappy as clinicians in discharging young patients with a sight-threatening condition over which we can do nothing, it is usual to follow these patients up at some arbitrary interval to monitor growth. However, strictly speaking, if the diagnosis is clear, this isn't really needed from a medical perspective, though might be justifiable from a diplomatic or political standpoint.

By far, the main reason that choroidal osteoma is mentioned here is the very high rate; one-third of patients, or more really, develop a secondary CNVM. Whilst osteomas alone are usually associated with a slow, gradual loss of vision, should a neovascular membrane develop, the vision, as expected, would start rapidly declining with marked blurring and distortion should the macula become involved. Examination reveals an osteoma plus fluid and blood, and the OCT and OCT-A are so predictable and mirror what we have seen before, so this will not be mentioned here. Again, treatment is the same as for any CNVM should the macula be threatened. However, if the membrane is away from the macula, it might pose no threat to vision and can be observed for long enough that the clinician can be reasonably certain that for now at least, no developing threat is present, and the patient can be discharged with home monitoring advice and the ubiquitous and dubiously helpful Amsler grid. Patients without CNVM present should be warned of the risk of developing it and again advised to monitor their eyes closely.

Christiana Says...

The enhanced-depth imaging OCT (EDI-OCT) can be a useful aid in confirming the presence of choroidal osteoma, demonstrating a characteristic lamellar (multiple hyperreflective lines with occasional denser lines) within the choroidal lesion (3). Anti-VEGF therapy tends to be very efficacious in CNVM secondary to choroidal osteoma, although ongoing treatment is typically required.

IATROGENIC SECONDARY NEOVASCULAR MEMBRANES

The main iatrogenic cause of secondary membrane development is the application of laser therapy to the retina as a result of conditions such as diabetes, retinal vein occlusion or indeed any ischaemic insult. The purpose of retinal laser is to intentionally damage the RPE and surrounding structures to prevent progression of the disease and added ischaemic damage to the eye via VEGF release and new vessel development at the disc, iris or elsewhere. In the case of panretinal photocoagulation (PRP), the laser scars are usually (well, should be) away from the macula. Any choroidal neovascularisation that may develop through a laser scar should be far enough away from the macula that no real action need to be taken apart from observation, with bleeding and ultimately scarring taking place to mark the end of the process in a form of controlled explosion, not too dissimilar to that seen in an eccentric disciform. Should fluid and blood creep too close to the macula for comfort, the decision-making process is reasonably simple because the only tool we have in our armamentarium capable of making a change is anti-VEGF injections. The regime should, of course, be the same as before; there is no need to add confusion by changing things around needlessly.

Whilst PRP scars are numerous, they are peripheral, and the risk posed to vision should a secondary CNVM develop is consequently low. Laser burns of far greater risk are found with focal laser, where the macula is intentionally targeted, and the fovea is avoided to reduce fluid leakage. The number of burns here and the power used are a lot less, but the location makes the consequences of membrane development much more serious and the chances of needing anti-VEGF therapy are much higher. Thankfully, the actual frequency of this complication occurring is very low anyhow and with focal laser now being almost, though not completely, replaced by injections it is not something that we need to worry about as much as in the past. Photodynamic therapy is also a risk factor for secondary membrane development. However, the rates of this being done are now almost nil, partly as a result of the inexplicable and scandalous increase in the price of verteporfin (late-stage capitalism) and partly because of newer therapies being available, the risk is nowhere near as much of a concern as before.

Lastly, patients will sometimes decide to shine a laser pointer pen into their own eyes or the eyes of their friends for no reason other than (pun intended) blind curiosity. Even though these laser pens are freely available to be purchased by the general public, unlike an Argon retinal laser machine for example, they are still very damaging to the eye and can leave a chorioretinal scar following traversal of the laser light beam across the retina, much like the laser seen in the James Bond film. Any mystery scar on the retina that resembles a worm or a snake could well be due to laser pen exposure. On top of the obvious potential damage to vision that the burn itself can cause, the development of secondary CNVM can make the result of a few moments of indiscretion (or bad luck) downright catastrophic. Patients can and do conceal the true history of having done such a stupid thing to themselves, so be wary if the tracks look typical and have a low index of suspicion, especially if the patient looks shifty when you mention laser pens. Again, should the exudation threaten the fovea and vision, the same anti-VEGF regime as used above and should always be used.

CENTRAL SEROUS CHORIORETINOPATHY

Central serous chorioretinopathy (CSCR) will be discussed in far more detail in Chapter 8 but is mentioned here as well because a secondary neovascular membrane can develop as a result. In a nutshell, CSCR is a condition in which the RPE is degraded by various mechanisms and fluid can collect transiently under the retina, causing symptoms. Every time the retina floods like this, the structure and function of both photoreceptors and RPE is affected in the same way that repeated flooding and drying of an electricity junction box would eventually start to degrade its function, cause short circuits and eventually cause it to fail altogether. The RPE and Bruch's complex are like the natural waterproofing layer of the eye and increasing degradation leads to cracks, and leaks can develop through those tracks.

Fundus autofluorescence (FAF) is a key investigation tool in CSCR, as it shows all sorts of hidden damage that's been done to the RPE over the years (see Chapter 8). It might be no surprise, therefore, that one of the longer-term dangers is that a neovascular complex can take advantage and grow through. The best advice is to

TABLE 5.2

Features of CNVM Secondary to CSCR on Multimodal Imaging

OCT	OCT-A	FFA	ICGA
Double-layer sign (shallow separation between the RPE and Bruch's membrane) – suggestive, not diagnostic Irregular pigment epithelial detachment	Flow signal highlighting that the PED is vascularised	CNVM detection can be poor due to chronic RPE changes.	Hyperfluorescent plaque or hot spot in late ICGA (10–15 minutes)

have a low index of suspicion, and if the nature of the fluid changes, not to assume automatically that this is just 'recurrent' disease. If there is intraretinal fluid development, and especially if there is blood present, OCT-A should be performed, and if a membrane is present, then anti-VEGF treatment should be instituted again the same as before. Do not reinvent the wheel!

Christiana Says...

Numerous studies have reported higher CNVM detection rates with OCT-A than FAF or a combination of FAF and indocyanine green angiography (ICGA) in the context of CSCR. However, OCT-A is not without pitfalls in this context due to segmentation errors, projection artefacts and the distorted RPE architecture in CSCR. When CNVM is suspected in these eyes, multimodal imaging incorporating OCT, OCT-A, and ICGA is helpful (see Table 5.2).

CNVM SECONDARY TO ANGIOID STREAKS

Angioid streaks are bilateral breaks in a weakened Bruch's membrane, radiating and branching irregularly from the optic disc. As with any break in Bruch's, these streaks can lead to secondary neovascularization, and though it is considered particularly aggressive and recurrent compared to other secondary CNVMs, the treatment is the same – namely, treat and extend anti-VEGF injections. Angioid streaks, which are 'streaks resembling blood vessels', can be associated with systemic conditions such that useful acronyms like PEPSI are remembered for exam purposes to help us remember the cause. In this case, P stands for the genetic condition pseudoxanthoma elasticum, E stands for Ehlers–Danlos syndrome, the other P stands for Paget's disease, S stands for sickle cell anaemia, and I for idiopathic (see below). CNVM secondary to angioid streaks can be difficult to treat, requiring frequent injections and prone to scarring. The streaks can be missed, so it is worth reviewing diagnostic images and the medical history of patients requiring frequent injections for possibly missed angioid streaks.

IDIOPATHIC NEOVASCULAR MEMBRANES

Idiopathic is derived from the same root as 'idiot' and simply means that the cause of something is unknown. In reality, of course, everything happens for a reason, with membrane development being no exception, but sometimes we just can't ever work out what that reason is. As mentioned before, any weakness, defect, or damage to the RPE–Bruch's complex increases the chance of choroidal neovascularisation and secondary membrane development. This might be due to some peculiar previously unrecognised congenital defect, some design flaw, or perhaps a moment too long spent staring at an eclipse, the sun, or some other bright light with that memory now long forgotten. Perhaps an unrecognised and undiagnosed condition caused a scar that then went on to develop problems years down the line such as toxoplasmosis, traumatic damage or something else again.

At the end of the day, it matters not what caused the issue. Presumably, whatever caused the insult has long stopped and is no longer relevant, although if this is not the case, then obviously things are different. However, in that case the membrane is not really idiopathic, it's just that you're not looking hard enough for the cause. A neovascular membrane is a neovascular membrane at the end of the day, and diagnosis and treatment is almost always the same anyhow. So, to summarise this chapter, if a membrane is present from whatever cause and is threatening vision, then inject, inject, inject.

Christiana Says...

This chapter underlines the value of careful diagnostic enquiry. Whilst the treatment is often the same, at least initially, the burden and prognosis is often different depending on the underlying cause.

REFERENCES

1. Wolf S, Balciuniene VJ, Laganovska G, Menchini U, Ohno-Matsui K, Sharma T, Wong TY, Silva R, Pilz S, Gekkieva M; RADIANCE Study Group. RADIANCE: A randomized controlled study of ranibizumab in patients with choroidal neovascularization secondary to pathologic myopia. Ophthalmology. 2014; 121(3):682–692.e2.
2. Ikuno Y, Ohno-Matsui K, Wong TY, Korobelnik JF, Vitti R, Li T, Stemper B, Asmus F, Zeitz O, Ishibashi T; MYRROR Investigators. Intravitreal aflibercept injection in patients with myopic choroidal neovascularization: The MYRROR study. Ophthalmology. 2015; 122(6):1220–1227.
3. Dinah C, Sandinha T. Enhanced depth imaging as an adjunctive tool in the diagnosis of decalcified choroidal osteoma. Eye (Lond). 2014; 28(3):356–358. doi: 10.1038/eye.2013.272. Epub 2014 Jan 10.

6 Diabetic Retinopathy and Maculopathy

There is an epidemic of diabetes affecting the world at present, with more than 8% of the population of the fair city of Swansea suffering from diabetes and 20% of the Welsh population either being diabetic or pre-diabetic. These figures, bad as they are, are worse again amongst some populations around the world. Individuals of African and South Asian descent have a twofold risk of visual impairment, severe visual impairment and loss of driving vision.

Obesity and diet are largely to blame for this, and poverty and economics are to blame for this in turn because it is type 2 diabetes that has exploded in incidence, not type 1. In some populations, there may well be a genetic predilection and a lot of work is ongoing to untangle this, especially given the exponential rise in young type 2 diabetes (type 2 diabetes developing before age 39). For all the complexity of diabetic eye disease, this can be summarised as 'does this patient need laser, anti–vascular endothelial growth factor (anti-VEGF) or steroid injections, both or none?' There is a lot of over-engineering when it comes to diabetic eye disease, with many books written on the most nuanced aspects of the condition that even then, might not come to any firm conclusions. Preventing sight loss and blindness in this patient population is ultimately a very rewarding endeavour.

TYPE 1 AND TYPE 2 DIABETES

There are myriad 'types' of diabetes, but this is an iteration of the famous coastline paradox, and ultimately, it's all a matter of perspective. For us simple ophthalmologists, there are just types 1 and 2 of any real interest. All others, such as gestational diabetes and diabetes related to genetic causes, can be forced into one of these two categories. Type 1 is related to failure of insulin production and patients tend to be young when diagnosed and otherwise well, whilst type 2 diabetes occurs due to people over time stressing their body with poor diet and lack of exercise. Although they do produce insulin, it becomes less potent over time, like an overworked clerk might become when faced with a gradually but inexorably increasing workload. Papers and files pile up unprocessed as the inbox keeps getting filled faster and faster. There is (as with everything) a genetic element at play here as well. Patients tend to be older and fatter, but not always. It is undoubtedly the case that lifestyle and such factors play a role in the development of type 2 diabetes that makes it a little bit more socially problematic to admit to having it, and with half of patients with type 2 diabetes requiring insulin on top of their other medication, usually biguanides such as metformin, it is not uncommon for type 2 patients to try and 'relabel' themselves as type 1. Be cautious of this.

DOI: 10.1201/9781003628309-6

For us simple ophthalmologists, the type of diabetes present is only of interest in determining how it progresses. Some younger type 1 diabetics go through a phase of teenaged rebellion, don't take their medication properly, and eventually when they calm down and mature, it is paradoxically and cruelly then and only then that the true nature of the disease catches up with them and things deteriorate. Other times, people try their best to maintain meticulous control and still fail. The worsening eye condition seen in diabetes is a bit like the unemployment rate and the economy. We might see stock market crashes on the news and plummeting FTSE100 and Dow Jones figures, but it takes months or even years for the effects to be felt with a rising unemployment rate, and consequently an improving economy takes a while to start employing people again. The swings are larger and can be much more devastating with type 1 diabetes, and the eye can become very damaged as a consequence.

Type 2 patients, on the other hand, tend to be older and less fit generally and are more likely to suffer from hypertension, heart disease and other such conditions. Not always, however, and perhaps not even mostly. Gestational diabetes can be seen as a potential harbinger of future type 2 diabetes, as the baby puts a strain on the body that eases after birth. The degree of eye disease present tends to be less devastating much of the time, but not always, and there is perhaps a higher incidence of patients not looking after their health, attending appointments regularly or listening to doctors. These are only rules of thumb, though. It is the explosion in type 2 diabetes that caused this diabetic tsunami facing eyecare services, and it is perhaps the case that new weight loss medications such as the new glucagon-like peptide 1 agonists can turn the tide by reducing appetites, and as such overeating, and as such type 2 diabetes. It is an exciting time.

We must remember that the human eye is also connected to the rest of the body, and diabetes has many effects – kidney disease, peripheral neuropathy and vasculopathy amongst many others. Both type 1 and type 2 diabetes can also cause death if the glucose is mismanaged, though this is a much greater danger with type 1. It is good to be aware of this if a diabetic patient is behaving oddly in clinic; don't just assume an awkward personality, dementia or such, and do not hesitate to do a blood glucose test if there is doubt (which could be very low or very high). With regard to general diabetes, though, the only duty we have as eyecare specialists is to advise smoking cessation, good diabetic control, eating and exercise habits, and being aware of extreme fluctuations in glucose so we can advise a responsible adult to help get things under control again. With regard to type 1 diabetes, this tends to be (but is not always so) a hospital diabetologist, and with type 2 diabetes, the general practitioner, both with an army of non-medical practitioners.

It is good to know that HbA1c levels are meant to be below 48 mmol/mol in regular patients, though 58 mmol/mol is tolerated instead if the patient is prone to hypoglycaemia. It is also good to know HbA1c levels as a general barometer of control, *but* it is absolutely *not* for us to mess around with diabetic medication ourselves. This is the purview of others, and too many cooks can not only spoil the broth but can end up poisoning it. We are not experts in the control of general diabetes and should we be concerned at the control, write a letter to their clinician and do not be tempted under any circumstances to fiddle around in an area that is outside your area of expertise.

Christiana Says...

High blood sugar (hyperglycemia) is toxic to the retinal blood vessels, resulting in the clinical features we describe as diabetic retinal disease. Low blood sugar (hypoglycaemia) is also dangerous, as is fluctuating sugar. However, hyperglycemia is also toxic to the retinal neurons. Therefore, diabetic retinal disease is not just a retinal vascular disease but rather a neurovascular disease of the retina. The availability of optical coherence tomography (OCT) has enabled more insights into how hyperglycemia affects retina tissue, and the functional impact of hyperglycemia is an area of extensive research. What is now established is that hyperglycemia affects the retinal neurons well ahead of the retinal vessels, this impact being evident earlier than the traditional features of diabetic retinal disease.

Emerging evidence shows several functional and structural changes precede clinically detectable diabetic retinopathy. These include peripapillary retinal nerve fibre layer thinning, reduced combined retinal ganglion cell layer and inner plexiform layer thickness on OCT prior to onset of clinically detectable diabetic retinopathy. These findings, known as diabetic retinal neurodegeneration, are thought to be a consequence of subclinical ischaemia and possibly the direct consequence of hyperglycemia on the retinal nerve fibre layer. This is important because current management strategies are often targeted at the vascular component of diabetic retinal disease. In the future, therapies that are directed at neuroprotection may be able to prevent the development of diabetic retinopathy in the first place.

DIABETIC RETINAL DISEASE

Glucose is poisonous to the body in the same way that oxygen is. It drives reactions and causes excess speed and therefore accidents to occur. The Deepwater Horizon film features a well blowout scene taking place, and highlights how gas entering the general intake causes lights to burn brighter and turbines to turn quicker in the buildup to the explosion itself. In the eye, the glucose drives reactions through inflammatory cascades that result in several issues: weakening of blood vessel walls, outpouchings in the form of microaneurysms (with their being 'micro' as a result of their being smaller in diameter than a retinal vein at the disc margin), macroaneurysms (to a much lesser degree), cotton wool spots (also termed soft exudates and due to ruptured axons in the nerve fibre layer spilling their axoplasmic interiors all over the immediate vicinity as a result of ischaemia), and hard exudates (lipids leaking from leaky blood vessels and settling at the edge of a flood like the grimy scum you get around the end of a bath). Dot and blot haemorrhages occur as blood vessels block and burst. Figure 6.1 illustrates the various features seen in diabetic eye disease and how they look to the clinician. The end result of all this damage is that capillaries, and later on, larger blood vessels, become leaky resulting in accumulation of fluid and lipid-rich deposits at the macular. Across the retina, blood flow is impeded resulting in impaired delivery of oxygen and nutrients to the retina decrease, and cells gradually starve. Areas of ischaemia occur as capillaries block off and VEGF and other cytokines are released by dying starved cells result in retinal neovascularisation, or on the iris, which does not in any way address the oxygenation issue. These new vessels, which grow on the surface of the retina using

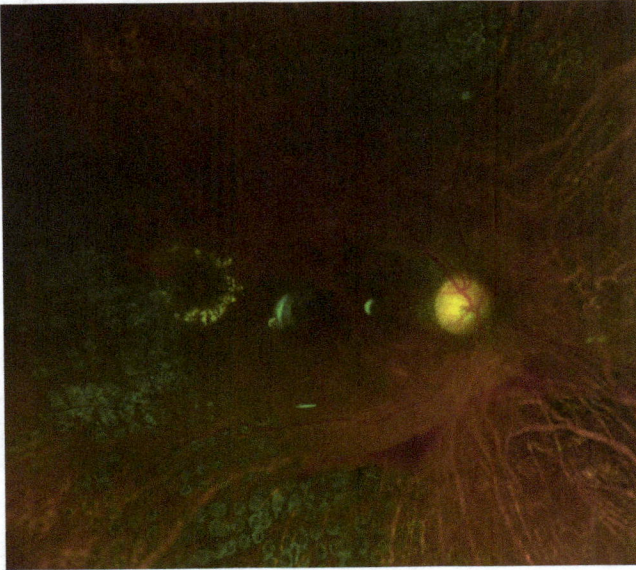

FIGURE 6.1   Diabetic eye disease.

the posterior vitreous base as an anchor, are weak, and do not have tight junctions; they are therefore liable to spontaneously bleed, leading to vitreous haemorrhage and sight loss. They also incorporate fibrous elements, which can pull on the retina, resulting in tractional retinal detachments.

Quite the contrary, in fact, new vessel growth is uncoordinated and does not address the problem; growth is haphazard, untidy and appears like a delicate sea anemone with fragile blood vessels just waiting to break. The optic disc is a common site for new vessel development, mainly because it is relatively fertile ground for VEGF to act. Figure 6.2 illustrates how new vessels at the disc (NVD) appear. If the VEGF dissipates to the front of the eye and reaches the iris, florid neovascularisation can occur here too. This is called 'rubeosis iridis' with rubeosis simply meaning 'red'. The iris looks red due to the presence of multiple blood vessels, though nowadays due to diabetic screening systems and hospital follow-up appointments, it is rare to see the whole iris red with blood vessels and a few twirls of twisty clumps is what is usually seen. Figure 6.3 illustrates how new vessels at the iris (NVI) look. New vessels can appear elsewhere around the retina as well, usually at the junction of ischaemic and non-ischaemic retina, sometimes in multiple variably sized configurations around the unseen ischaemic border. These vessels are somewhat appropriately called new vessels elsewhere (NVE). Figure 6.4 illustrates the appearance of NVE.

There are consequences to this new vessel growth. Vessels lead to bleeding and bleeding leads to scarring. At the iris, the NVI cause gradual scarring where the iris starts to zipper shut the trabecular meshwork, termed anterior synechiae (as opposed to the posterior synechiae seen on the posterior surface of the iris in uveitis), with predictable effects on interocular pressure. The form of glaucoma that occurs with

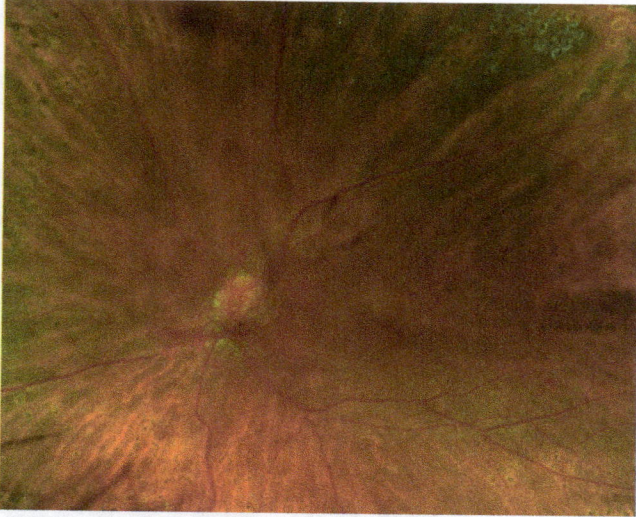

FIGURE 6.2   New vessels at the disc (NVD).

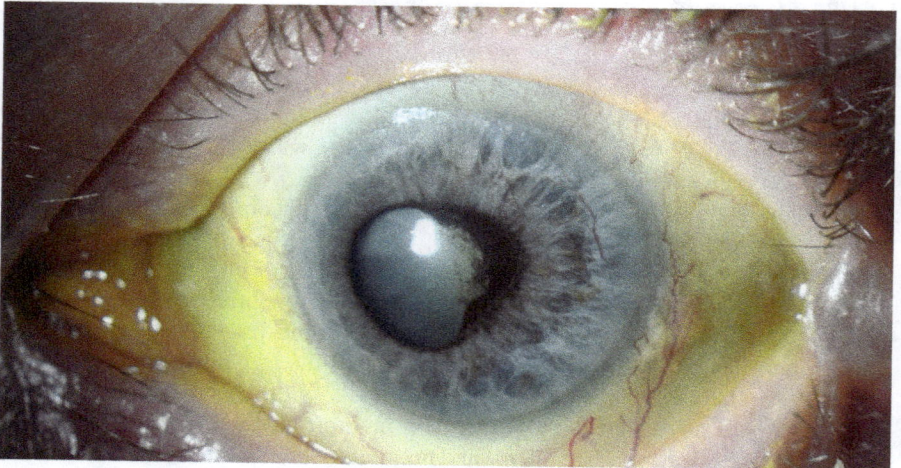

FIGURE 6.3   New vessels at the iris (NVI).

unchecked untreated NVI is termed 'neovascular glaucoma' and brings dismay to both Medical Retina specialists and glaucoma surgeons alike. The name of the game so far as well are concerned is to spot this development early and treat the patient quickly enough that the horrendous intractable pressure problems that lead to blindness are avoided. Once you reach the stage of a fully zipped shut angle, it is a very difficult situation to recover from.

NVD or NVE do not affect pressure, but can do one of two things: fill up the eye with blood or cause a tractional retinal detachment. Patients sometimes report

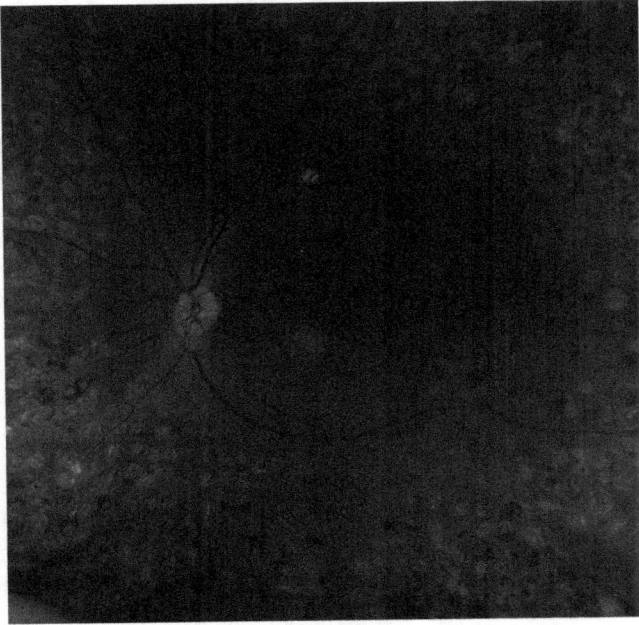

FIGURE 6.4 New vessels elsewhere (NVE).

showers of floaters in the run-up to a proper vitreous haemorrhage, which can cause vision to plummet to nothing in the space of a few hours. Sometimes the haemorrhaging is more insidious and builds up slowly, never fully filling the eye with blood. Blood is a hugely gliogenic fluid and leads to scarring in a futile attempt for the body to stop the blood flow. With the eye, the scarring process leads to an epiretinal membrane at the most benign end of the scale, increasing to areas of traction that extend from new vessel tufts to surrounding retina, gradually pulling and pulling until a tractional retinal detachment occurs. Figure 6.5 demonstrates a tractional

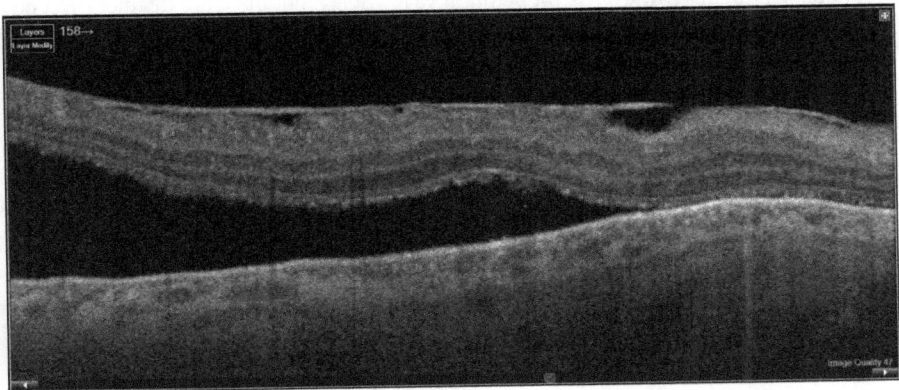

FIGURE 6.5 Tractional retinal detachment in diabetic eye disease.

retinal detachment in the context of diabetic eye disease. This tractional detachment can then lead to a rhegmatogenous detachment because the ratcheting of the tension results in a retinal break, and then at the worst end of the scale, the whole retina can come away resulting in a total detachment that is so scarred it cannot be replaced. But this is not the worst situation. Sometimes, although rarely, uncontrolled pressure issues with this now blind eye can cause so many problems for the patient; pain, uveitis and so on, that removal of the eye is the only option left.

There are many other effects that diabetes can have on the eye, though because these are so numerous but decreasingly important, it is not useful to know more than the above about how diabetic eye disease presents. The next challenge is working out how to work up and treat diabetic retinopathy and maculopathy.

PRESENTATION

The vast majority of patients presenting to the eye department already have a diagnosis of diabetes and have, in fact, been referred via a screening system such as Diabetic Eye Screening Wales (DESW) or any other local variant. Some will have been referred by optometrists and others, again, from diabetologists or general practitioners because of ocular concerns. Most patients with diabetic eye disease have no symptoms at all and can come across as incredulous and unbelieving when told that they have a serious issue with their eye that if left unaddressed will threaten vision. Others might be severe enough that they have actually started to experience symptoms such as blurring, dark patches, distortion or phenomena such as minification in the case of maculopathy or floaters in the form of cobwebs or strings in the case of retinopathy.

It is extremely rare in Wales, Britain and the rest of Europe, despite our increasingly dysfunctional health service, for patients to present with advanced diabetic eye disease with retinal detachment. Neovascular glaucoma, on the other hand, is a bellwether of how safe the appointment system is, as delayed appointments, such as occurred during the COVID-19 outbreak, resulted in a significant increase in cases with a subsequent decrease in recovery. Symptoms here are pain and vision loss, such as would occur during an attack of angle closure glaucoma.

Patients' attitudes towards their condition vary widely, but there are distinct subtypes under the umbrella of diabetic eye disease. There are concerned patients with minimal symptoms that cannot be explained by any investigation, who often present because they are worried about their vision. There are patients with poorly controlled disease who battle hard to try to control things and with whom you share many of the ups and downs of life and whom you get to know well. Perhaps the most difficult types, though, fall into two other categories: First, the patients who pay their condition little heed as they are mostly asymptomatic and frequently do not attend (DNA) appointments or take any personal responsibility in controlling their diabetes, instead devolving all responsibility to healthcare providers. The second is the evolution of this first type, where their disease has caught up with them and their vision is damaged as a result; they are usually in need of injections, laser or both, and vociferously complain about a perceived lack of improvement in symptoms and blame various healthcare agencies for their condition, including your good self, instead of taking any personal responsibility. It is important to be aware of this phenomenon so their corrosive attitudes do not distract you from your valuable work in saving sight; as Samuel Shem says, 'the patient is the one with the disease'.

Christiana Says...

From a public health perspective, a significant proportion of diabetes-related vision loss can be prevented through a systems-level approach that includes targeted education, community-level or national diabetic retinopathy screening with timely referral pathways for further investigation, monitoring or treatment. The UK has a world-leading, centrally funded diabetic retinopathy screening programme, with the English programme providing annual screening for over 3.3 million eligible people with diabetes aged 12 and above. Primary care clinicians refer everyone newly diagnosed to the screening programme for screening within 3 months. Similar programmes operate in Scotland, Wales and Northern Ireland. Although general uptake of screening is high (>80% in England in 2018/2019), this overall figure masks suboptimal attendance in particular demographics (adults <35 years, lower socioeconomic status and mixed ethnicity groups as an example). Another study reported that the annual incidence of new certifications for vision impairment in young adults (<35 years) failed to show the net decline that has occurred in other age groups between 2009 and 2019. In addition, there is good evidence that the more diabetic eye screening appointments are missed, the greater the risk that the next attendance will reveal sight-threatening disease.

Extensive work has been conducted to understand the barriers to attendance of screening appointments in vulnerable groups, and the major factors appear to be the lack of integration of retinopathy screening with other processes of diabetes care, challenges accessing screening services and difficulties with scheduling appointments. In my view, at the core, is the lack of integration of voices from these groups in the design of screening services. Diabetes is a multiorgan disease, often affecting all areas of an individual's life, including social, psychological, and economic aspects in addition to the physical impact. Clinicians looking after diabetic retinal disease need to remain aware of the whole patient connected to the eye and the ecosystem within which they have to manage their eye disease.

DIAGNOSIS AND GRADING OF SEVERITY

As mentioned in the previous section, the diagnosis of diabetes is almost always already made long before the patient ever reaches you. Every so often, however, though it is extremely rare even still, you will come across undiagnosed diabetes yourself. This is usually in the context of patients presenting with perhaps a retinal vein occlusion (RVO), macroaneurysm or unexplained haemorrhages at the fundus where blood tests have been ordered, including glucose and potentially an HbA1c. If diabetes is detected, then write a letter to their general practitioner to properly take over care and initiate treatment; there is no role for the ophthalmologist in treating diabetes itself.

Helpfully, however, this is unusual, and the diagnosis is made for you, though it must always be remembered that though the patient suffers from diabetes, not everything affecting their eyes might be due to diabetic eye disease. The inverse of the above is that patients with diabetes are at increased risk of RVO and hypertension, for example, and so it is always useful to consider alternate or ancillary diagnoses. Ocular ischaemic syndrome is another ischaemic eye condition that looks like diabetic eye disease, but instead of diabetes being responsible, the narrowing of the carotid is the cause. In fact, anything that causes ischaemia can mimic diabetic eye disease as ultimately ischaemia is the end result of a number of phenomena; radiation retinopathy, for example.

It is important to bear this in mind so that an index of suspicion is maintained for patients who are slightly unusual. If the disease is very asymmetric, for example, it is useful to consider ocular ischaemic syndrome. If the amount of haemorrhaging in an eye is significantly worse in one quadrant, could a branch RVO be present on top of the diabetes? If there is a history of radiotherapy to the eye, could it be radiation-related damage rather than diabetes? Whilst in reality these situations are not that common, they are important to bear in mind so that extra tests can be ordered, such as blood pressure measurements or carotid Dopplers.

Never ever assume that just because a patient is referred with diabetes that diabetes alone is the cause of all their ocular ills.

Once it has been satisfactorily determined that diabetic retinopathy is indeed present and responsible for the current eye disease, its severity must then be graded. There are multiple different ways if doing this, and whilst the Welsh method will be presented here, it is important to find out what system your country or local area employs and stick to that. The Welsh grading system is separated into Retinopathy (R) and Maculopathy (M). Table 6.1 demonstrates what the grading means.

Each eye will be given an R and an M rating, with U being reserved for eyes where the details cannot be seen with enough detail to properly determine what the grading is, perhaps due to a cataract or some other media opacity. In a practical sense, it is easier to determine the grading by following these rules, starting with R and then following on to M:

Step 1: Is the eye totally normal? If so, it is R0.
Step 2: If it is not normal, is there any proliferative disease present? NVI, NVD or NVE? If so, has it been treated in the past with panretinal photocoagulation (PRP) laser and is it now no longer bleeding and growing? If so, it is R3S.
Step 3: If it's newly discovered neovascularisation, is it definitely new and is it definitely untreated? If so, it is R3A.

TABLE 6.1
Grading of Diabetic Retinopathy and Maculopathy

Grading	Meaning
R0	No retinopathy present
R1	Background diabetic retinopathy
R2	Pre-proliferative diabetic retinopathy
R3A	Active proliferative diabetic retinopathy
R3S	Stable proliferative diabetic retinopathy
M0	No maculopathy present
M1A	Active maculopathy present
M1S	Stable maculopathy present
U	Ungradable

Step 4: If the eye is neither normal nor proliferative but has retinopathy present, does it fulfil the 4:2:1 rule? This refers to the presence in 4 quadrants of multiple blot haemorrhages, at least 2 quadrants of venous beading, or at least 1 quadrant containing intraretinal microvascular abnormalities (IRMA; twisty blood vessels that look like and mimic new vessels but aren't new vessels and don't bleed). If so, then it is R2. If not, it is R1.
Step 5: Is there maculopathy present? If not, it is M0.
Step 6: If there is maculopathy present, does it need any treatment or is it stable? If the former, it is M1A, and if the latter, M1S. Treatment will be discussed below.

The aim of grading severity is simply to work out how to manage and follow up the patient. Treatment takes place only for R3A and M1A eyes.
Christiana Says...
To move forward, it is often important to understand where we have been. In the mid-20th century, diabetic retinopathy was being increasingly recognized as a serious complication of diabetes, but there was no universally accepted way to describe the stages and severity, which made it very difficult to compare studies, identify which patients needed treatment or track disease progression. To solve this, a group of leading retinal specialists, diabetologists and researchers convened at the Airlie House conference centre in Virginia in 1968, sponsored by the National Eye Institute and other research bodies. The ambitious goal was to create a comprehensive, standardized, classification system of diabetic retinopathy that would be useful in both clinical care and research. The participants catalogued specific retinal findings and then created a grading scale that captured the progression from mild to severe disease.

The Airlie House classification became the foundation for the Early Treatment Diabetic Retinopathy Study (ETDRS) – a massive, National Institutes of Health (NIH)-sponsored clinical trial in the 1980s that continues to influence practice to this day (see Table 6.2). This led to the ETDRS severity scale, modern screening and

TABLE 6.2
ETDRS Severity Scale

ETDRS Scale

10	Diabetic retinopathy absent
20	Microaneurysms only
35	Mild non-proliferative diabetic retinopathy (NPDR)
43	Moderate NPDR
47	Moderately severe NPDR
53	Severe or very severe NPDR
60	Scars of photocoagulation for proliferative diabetic retinopathy (PDR)
61	Mild PDR
65	Moderate PDR
71, 75	High risk PDR

treatment guidelines, and evidence-based recommendations for laser photocoagulation and later anti-VEGF therapy.

TREATMENT

There are two aspects here: when to treat and how to treat. A third consideration then concerns special circumstances, but let us take each aspect in turn.

WHEN TO TREAT

There are many guidelines written about this issue, but they are just that – guides. First principles dictate 'primum non nocere' – first do no harm. Finding abnormalities does not mean that something needs to be done just for the sake of doing something. Let us start with retinopathy and then move on to maculopathy. The main reason we see patients with diabetes is to detect neovascularisation at an early stage where treatment can make a difference. If patients have either R0 or R1 disease, they can be safely discharged from a retinopathy perspective back to DESW or a local variant. There is no business in precious but scarce hospital eye appointments being used up looking at such minimal disease. Annoyingly, but not that infrequently, nervous people in primary care or outside medical retina will detect signs of diabetic eye disease, albeit very mild, and send the patient in as the eye 'has retinopathy'. This is where education of colleagues is just so very important.

R2 disease looks worse than R1, obviously, but even still, there is only very rarely a need to treat this. In most cases, monitoring is best; writing letters at each appointment to the general practitioner or diabetologist so they know if the eye is improving or deteriorating. The safest gap between appointments is 3 months, but up to 6 monthly appointments can be justified here, either face-to-face or via a virtual clinic system. If the local environment has suitably trained medical retina-qualified optometrists in primary care, such as exist in Wales, then this is another option to save precious hospital capacity from being wasted. A case could conceivably be made for treating patients with very significant R2 pre-proliferative disease if the patient's control is very poor and attendance very patchy. If the patient is perhaps expected to deteriorate from a medical perspective and not be in a position to undergo laser therapy in the near future, a case can be made if pre-proliferative disease is expected to worsen. However, the default is to watch.

Christiana Says...

The ETDRS laid the foundations for how and when patients with diabetic retinopathy are treated to prevent vision loss. This study, which started in 1979, recruited 3711 patients with mild to severe non-proliferative diabetic retinopathy (NPDR) or early proliferative diabetic retinopathy (PDR) and sort to determine when treatment should begin, whether early treatment prevents progression to vision-threatening PDR and the role of aspirin therapy in managing diabetic retinopathy. They found that early PRP in eyes with high-risk PDR (see Table 6.3) resulted in a 50% reduction in the risk of severe vision loss at 5 years (severe vision loss was defined as best corrected visual acuity [BCVA] 5/200 at two consecutive visits 4 months apart). This was the evidence that made prompt PRP the standard of care for high-risk PDR. Indeed, these days, we don't tend to wait for high-risk PDR, with PRP being offered to most

TABLE 6.3
Definition of High-Risk PDR

High-Risk PDR

1. Neovascularization of the disc (NVD) ≥ ¼ to 1/3 disc area in size with or without vitreous or preretinal haemorrhage
2. **Any size NVD with** vitreous or preretinal hemorrhage
3. **Neovascularization elsewhere (NVE) ≥ 1/2 disc area with** vitreous or preretinal hemorrhage

patients on development of PDR as they typically progress without treatment. In summary, intravitreal anti-VEGF therapies perform just as well as intravitreal anti-VEGF studies; Clarity and Protocol S and DRCR.net study surgery versus injection

With the incredible results seen with anti-VEGF therapy for diabetic macular oedema (DMO), it was noted that retinal neovascularization tended to regress with these treatments as well. In clinical practice, intravitreal bevacizumab began to be frequently used to temporize PDR pending laser and as an adjunct to PRP. This led to clinical trials to determine whether anti-VEGF therapy is a suitable alternative to PRP. The results of two landmark studies on this topic are summarised in Table 6.4.

On the other hand, the vast majority of people with moderate and severe NPDR are observed. Preventing progression to PDR is desirable because PDR is associated with

TABLE 6.4
Protocol S and Clarity

	Protocol S	CLARITY
Intervention	Ranibizumab 0.5 mg dosed monthly X4 + PRN	Aflibercept 2 mg dosed monthly X3 + PRN
Comparator	PRP	PRP
No. of participants	394	232
Key eligibility criteria	1. Active PDR 2. No prior PRP 3. DMO allowed 4. Both eyes could be randomised	1. Active PDR 2. Could have had prior PRP but not more than 1 session 3. Only 1 eye randomized 4. No DMO requiring treatment
Primary outcome	Mean change in VA was comparable: +2.8 letters in ranibizumab arm vs +0.2 letters in PRP arm	Mean change in VA in the Aflibercept arm was +1.3 vs −2.9 in the PRP arm. Therefore, Aflibercept was both non-inferior and superior to PRP
Practice implications	• Ranibizumab is a viable treatment option for PDR. Visual field better preserved in this arm vs PRP arm. • However, at 5 years, over 1/3rd lost to follow-up	Aflibercept is a viable treatment option for PDR and provides superior statistically significant visual acuity gains. The study also demonstrated better binocular visual acuity and Esterman visual field scores.

a high risk of sight loss, and the gold standard treatment for PDR involves thermal destruction of the peripheral retina. However, the ETDRS study showed that early PRP in severe NPDR did reduce the risk of progressing to high-risk PDR and eventual severe vision loss, but the benefit was much smaller and there was a short-term drop in visual acuity in some eyes due to side effects of PRP. At 5 years, the risk of severe vision loss in this group was 4–6%, which decreased to 2–3% with PRP.

Like was done with PRP, more recent efforts have been made to evaluate anti-VEGF therapies for risk reduction in severe NPDR. The RISE and RIDE trials showed significant regression of diabetic retinopathy. These trials evaluated ranibizumab for DMO and included many eyes with concurrent severe NPDR and PDR and pre-specified Diabetic Retinopathy Severity Score (DRSS) analysis. This data led to U.S. Food and Drug Administration (FDA) approval of ranibizumab for diabetic retinopathy in patients with DMO, which was later broadened to all diabetic retinopathy.

Importantly, the Protocol W and PANORAMA studies, as seen in Table 6.5, evaluate severe NPDR. The sham arm of these studies reported progression rates to PDR of under 20% in 1 year contrasted with 50% in the sham arm of the ETDRS

TABLE 6.5
Summary of Key NPDR Studies

	Protocol W	PANORAMA
Intervention	Aflibercept 2 mg dosed monthly for 3 months, then 8-week intervals then every 16 weeks	Aflibercept 2 mg dosed monthly for 3 months, then 8-week intervals through 1 year
Comparator	Sham injection at the same schedule	Sham injection at the same schedule
No. of participants	399 eyes	402
Key eligibility criteria	Moderate to severe NPDR (ETDRS 43–53) No prior treatment for diabetic retinopathy Good visual acuity (6/7.5 or better) No PDR or centre-involving DMO at baseline	Same as Protocol W
Primary outcome	The endpoint was time to occurrence of either PDR or centre-involving DMO in the study eye. 16% developed the endpoint by 2 years in the Aflibercept arm vs 43% in the sham arm.	80% in the Aflibercept arm achieved a ≥ 2-step DRSS improvement vs 32% in the sham arm.
Practical implication	Although there was a reduction of risk of developing vision-threatening complications with Aflibercept, there was no difference in visual acuity in either arm at 2 years or at 4 years. The uptake of Aflibercept for NPDR is low even in regions where licensed for this reason.	Despite good anatomic results, lack of functional benefit has meant few clinicians treat severe NPDR with intravitreal anti-VEGF.

trials, likely due to the improved management of diabetes in recent cohorts. This underlines the importance of systemic management in diabetic retinopathy and the need to provide holistic care.

Despite the findings from the NPDR trials, the uptake for treatment is relatively low in countries where these treatments are licensed, and in the UK, there is really no uptake as these treatments are not funded by the National Institute for Health and Care Excellence (NICE). This is due to valid concerns about cost, treatment burden and associated risk of frequent intravitreal injections, loss of follow-up rates, and lack of true disease modification resulting in advanced presentation on re-presentation.

There is much enthusiasm and research interest evaluating fenofibrate for diabetic retinopathy. This came about from exploratory analysis of cardiovascular trials, the FIELD study (2007) and the ACCORD-EYE study (2010), which found that fenofibrate reduced the need for laser or slowed progression of diabetic retinopathy independent of lipid levels. As these were secondary endpoints, other dedicated studies have been set up to answer the question. The LENS study evaluated people with type 1 and type 2 diabetes and moderate NPDR in the Scottish national diabetic eye screening program and found that progression to referrable diabetic retinopathy or requirement for retinal laser, intravitreal injection or vitrectomy occurred in 22.7% of the fenofibrate arm versus 29.2% in the placebo arm, which is equivalent to a 27% risk reduction. Importantly, over 90% of participants had mild bilateral diabetic retinopathy, and as such, lower risk of progression. The NICE guidance for diabetic retinopathy recommends consideration of fenofibrate in people with referrable NPDR. More evidence for fenofibrate in diabetic retinopathy is expected from the DRCR.net Protocol AF study and the Australian FAME 1 study.

With R3 disease, the determination needs to be made as to whether it is active or not. Active disease implies new vessels in the presence of an untreated fundus (as in no laser has ever been applied) or new vessels that have documented growth between appointments despite previous treatment. These are then termed R3A patients and treatment should be considered the norm. In the past (and in some places today), determinations were made regarding how severe the R3A disease was based on the presence or absence of vitreous haemorrhage and the extent of the new vessel complex on the disc. In reality nowadays, any detection of definite new vessels should be grounds to consider laser treatment as appointments are not always reliable and neither are patients. A missed or delayed appointment can mean the difference between treating proliferative disease in time and missing the boat and ending up with an eye full of blood or a painful blind eye due to neovascular glaucoma. So unless there are extenuating circumstances, it is best to treat with laser.

These exceptions (and there are always exceptions) might include patients who have, in fact, had new vessels documented to be present for a long time without change, who were perhaps not properly diagnosed as new vessels in the past. These patients have a history of stability and as such, can perhaps be monitored and treated as R2 disease for practical purposes, though any change, however small, should mean laser, of course. Other exceptions might include patients with very minimal new vessel disease (especially if associated with minimal capillary non-perfusion), who are reliable sensible attenders but reticent to have laser unless absolutely needed, for whatever reason. In those cases, seeing them every 3 months and looking for any documented progression in their disease might be the best way forward, with progression equalling laser. However, with R3A disease, the default is treatment. R3S disease patients, by definition, have had a course of PRP, and because there is no documented progression of new vessels since laser was applied, they are, by definition, stable. They can be seen at increasing intervals, and if after extending intervals to 12 monthly, in 3 monthly steps, they are still stable, then discharge to the screening system can take place. There is no purpose in keeping R3S patients under the hospital if all is stable.

Let us now discuss maculopathy. M0 patients, by definition, have no maculopathy and can be passed back to the screening system. If maculopathy is present, it then needs to be determined if it is active and in need of treatment, M1A, or mild enough to be stable and not in need of treatment, M1S. Again, there are guidelines, but they are not hard-and-fast rules, and it is best to consider the patient at the centre of the decision-making progress. Unlike with proliferative retinopathy, the treatment for maculopathy isn't a well-defined course of a therapy that usually does not need to be repeated; injections normally carry on for a long time. Therefore, patients need to be fully on board with the plan for it to be successful. The first question to ask is, 'what symptoms, if any, have you had with your vision?' If patients report symptoms of maculopathy, as discussed above, then the visual acuity and degree of maculopathy need to be considered. If the vision is better than 0.18 on the LogMAR Chart (equivalent to 6/9 on the Snellen Chart), then regardless of the amount of fluid present, it is difficult to justify starting treatment in the absence of significant symptoms. The better the vision, the worse the symptoms need to be to justify starting injections, and there is no symptom complex that could arguably exist that would justify starting treatment in patients with vision of 0.00 LogMAR or better.

Considering the amount of fluid present is important as well, mainly as a determination must be made as to whether the fluid is to blame for the visual issues. Patients with diabetes have visual issues for all sorts of reasons: cataract, macular ischaemia, dry eye and many more. Traditionally, a thickness of 400 microns at the centre of the macula has been used as a cutoff for this based on NICE guidelines, but this is a soft cutoff. It is a guideline and not a law. It is still useful, however, as treating patients with visual issues not due to fluid with injections is not in the patient's best interest. So symptomatic patients with, say, 380 microns of fluid centrally should not be denied treatment for the sake of 20 microns, whilst similarly symptomatic patients with only a few parafoveal cysts and a thickness of 300 microns are unlikely to benefit.

Going the other way, if the vision is worse than 0.30 LogMAR (6/12 Snellen), then treatment can be justified even in the absence of any symptoms, again, if it is macular fluid itself, then that is to blame for the poor vision. Fluid has a deleterious effect on retinal function and over time marinating in fluid causes permanent dysfunction of the photoreceptor cells specifically and the retina in general. If the vision is worse than 0.30 LogMAR and the central thickness above 400 microns, then it is reasonable to conclude that the eye is suffering because of the fluid, and treatment is justified (and if the patient is agreeable of course) in the absence of actual symptoms. Funnily enough, as with any asymmetric medical retina disease, it is surprising how little patients can sometimes notice the vision deteriorate in one eye if there is good vision in the other.

If the vision is worse than 1.20 LogMAR (6/96 Snellen), then a soft border is reached when even though the vision is terrible and the fluid might be significant, treatment might not necessarily be in the patient's best interest. This is principally because it might not do anything, the horse has bolted so to speak, but again this is a guide. If the fluid is substantial and the vision close to the border, then it might be argued that if the patient is symptomatic, there is benefit in giving treatment a try, with a guarded prognosis and a proviso that should vision not improve, then treatment would be suspended. There are limits, though, and it could be argued that a patient with vision worse than 1.40 never be offered treatment and some sort of gradually diminishing sliding scale used between 1.20 and 1.40. There might even be circumstances where you'd give a one-off treatment if the vision was worse than 1.40 LogMAR just to test the water, but never if it is counting fingers (CF) or worse. Similarly, patients with vision better than 1.20 LogMAR might be better off avoiding treatment initiation if the changes present are chronic and the structure of the retina has already started to disintegrate on OCT scanning. We need to know our patient. This is where medicine becomes an art, and we realise ophthalmology is not a hard science. It gives us some hope that, even in the age of artificial intelligence (AI), our specific skill set means we will never be usurped.

Christiana Says...

The ETDRS study also had an arm that focused on establishing the definition of clinically significant macular oedema and its management. It found that in eyes with clinically significant macular oedema, focal/grid laser reduced the risk of moderate vision loss (defined as a doubling of the visual angle, i.e. three ETDRS lines) at 3 years by approximately 50% with some patients even gaining vision (see Table 6.6).

Laser treatment remained the gold standard for DMO for over 30 years. However, laser had limitations. It mainly stabilized vision rather than improved it, with some patients still experiencing progressive vision loss despite laser, and diffuse macular oedema involving the fovea particularly fared badly. Initially, due to mounting evidence of the role of inflammation and vascular leakage in DMO, periocular steroids were used in recalcitrant cases of DMO with some benefit. Early studies showed modest visual gains in these cases; however, there were increased rates of cataract progression, elevated intraocular pressure and short duration of action. Most importantly, steroids proved the proof of concept – pharmacologic suppression of oedema

TABLE 6.6
Definition of Clinically Significant Macular Oedema

1. **Retinal thickening** (oedema) at or within 500 microns (about 1/3 of a disc diameter) of the centre of the macula
2. Hard exudates at or within 500 microns of the centre of the macula, if associated with adjacent retinal thickening
3. Retinal thickening of one disc area (about 1500 microns in diameter) or larger, any part of which is within one disc diameter of the centre of the macula

could improve vision, unlike laser alone. Research in the 1990s identified VEGF as a key molecular driver mediating vascular permeability and contributing to retinal swelling and breakdown of the blood–retinal barrier, making targeted pharmacologic therapy plausible. The first licensed anti-VEGF therapy for DMO was ranibizumab, supported by the RISE and RIDE trial, which demonstrated 40–50% of patients gained 15 letters or more at 24 months versus 18% for sham (see Table 6.7).

How to Treat

PDR, whether NVD, NVE or NVI, is only really treated with retinal laser photocoagulation. The DRCR.net Protocol S famously determined that regular anti-VEGF injections were non-inferior to laser, which is academic-speak for just as good, but this is totally untenable in Wales, Europe and the real world. There is simply no capacity and no cash to keep injecting proliferative diabetic patients every month or two forever, without even mentioning the safety risks that would come as a result of patients being unable to attend for whatever reason, let alone the cumulative risks of 20,000 injections. Laser is the only way, and there are two ways to organise this; regular PRP and targeted PRP.

If a patient presents with NVD or NVE, then a course of PRP is in order. This should consist of 200-micron spots totalling at least 2500 spread over two sessions ideally, although it is oftentimes psychologically desirable for the ophthalmologist to break the back of the work and apply 1500 shots in the first session and then approximately 1000 in the second. With this approach, the patient is pleasantly surprised the second time rather than increasingly dismayed. A usual course on a pascal machine would include spots 10 ms in duration at a power of approximately 300–500 mW. You want a good reaction, what is termed an 'old-fashioned National Health Service (NHS) laser'. A nice white spot in a nice block grid of nine at a time. It is better to apply laser inferiorly first in case the vessels bleed between the first and second laser sessions and the inferior retina (for blood also follows Newtonian physics) will sink to the bottom before filling the top. It is better to draw the posterior border first with laser, just outside the arcades and a disc diameter nasal to the disc. Temporally, the same distance from the disc to the fovea outward again from the fovea should be used to mark the posterior temporal edge; unfortunately, it is far too common for ophthalmologists to leave a huge ellipse of unlasered retina stretching far too peripherally leaving a huge space of ischaemic retina leaking VEGF into the vitreous. Figure 6.6 demonstrates the ideal posterior border of the traditional PRP laser course.

Try not to leave large spaces, and fill equally in all directions. If the patient is squeamish and being difficult, by all means reduce the power slightly, reduce the box to a grid of four or even less and consider breaking the laser over three or even more sessions to make it easier, but do *not* under any circumstances leave the patient with inadequate treatment just because the whole thing is difficult and annoying. You will simply cause more problems for yourself and the patient down the line. It is better to overtreat than undertreat. Some people might argue that micropulse laser is just as good, that you can get away with fewer shots or that some combination of laser and anti-VEGF is good, but do not listen; to make a patient safe, the best treatment is good treatment.

TABLE 6.7
Summary of Pivotal Trials in DMO

	RISE and RIDE	VIVID and VISTA	Protocol T	MEAD1 and MEAD2	FAME	YOSEMITE and RHINE	PHOTON
Intervention	• Ranibizumab 0.3 mg monthly • Ranibizumab 0.5 mg monthly	Aflibercept 2 mg monthly × 5 and then every 4 weeks or every 8 weeks	Aflibercept 2 mg every 4 weeks to stabilisation + PRN	Ozurdex 0.35 mg at a minimum of 6-month intervals Or Ozurdex 0.7 mg at a minimum of 6-month intervals	0.2 µg/d Iluvien insert or 0.5 µg Iluvien	Faricimab dosed monthly × 4 and then personalised up to 16 weeks or Faricimab dosed monthly × 4 and then 8 weekly	Aflibercept 8 mg dosed monthly × 3 and then 12 weekly or 16 weekly
Comparator	Sham injections in the same schedule	Macular laser	Bevacizumab Ranibizumab Both dosed monthly till stabilisation + PRN	Sham	Sham	Aflibercept 2 mg monthly × 5 and then 8 weekly	Aflibercept 2 mg dosed monthly × 5 and then 8 weekly
No. of participants	759	872	660	1048	956	1891	660
Key eligibility criteria	• Centre-involving DMO • VA 6/12 or worse • Treatment-naive	• Centre-involving DMO • VA 6/12 or worse • Treatment-naïve and previously treated	Centre-involving DMO • VA 6/7.5 or worse	Centre-involving DMO • Previously treated • Treatment-naïve and not suitable for laser • VA 6/12 or worse	Centre-involving DMO At least 1 prior macular laser VA 6/12 or worse	Centre-involving DMO 6/12 or better Treatment-naïve or previously treated	Centre-involving DMO VA 6/7.5 or worse Treatment-naïve or previously treated

(Continued)

TABLE 6.7 (Continued)
Summary of Pivotal Trials in DMO

	RISE and RIDE	VIVID and VISTA	Protocol T	MEAD1 and MEAD2	FAME	YOSEMITE and RHINE	PHOTON
Primary outcome	40–44% gained ≥ 15 letters in the ranibizumab vs 18% in the sham arm	**Mean gain of 10.7 to 12.5 letters** at 52 weeks in the Aflibercept arm vs 0.9–1.7 letters in the laser arm	Mean gain of 13.3 with Aflibercept, +9.7 with bevacizumab and +11.2 with ranibizumab at 12 months Aflibercept performed much better than the other therapies in eyes with VA <6/18	**22.2% of high-dose Ozurdex-treated eyes and 18.4% of low-dose** Ozurdex-treated eyes gained ≥15 letters at 3 years vs 12% in the sham arm.	At month 36, 28.7% achieved ≥ 15 letters in the low-dose arm, 27.8% in the high-dose arm and 18.9% in the sham arm.	Faricimab arms gained 10–11 letters vs Aflibercept arm 10–11 letters	Mean gain +8.8 in the 8-mg 12-week arm, +7.9 in the 8-mg 16-week arm and +9.2 in the Aflibercept 2-mg arm
Practice implication	Established ranibizumab as a first-line therapy for DMO	Aflibercept superior to laser	All three effective but Aflibercept favoured in eyes with lower vision at baseline	Ozurdex efficacious in DMO especially in previously treated patients or unsuitable for anti-VEGF	Long-acting steroid effective for chronic DMO	Faricimab was non-inferior to Aflibercept	Aflibercept 8 mg was non-inferior to Aflibercept 2 mg

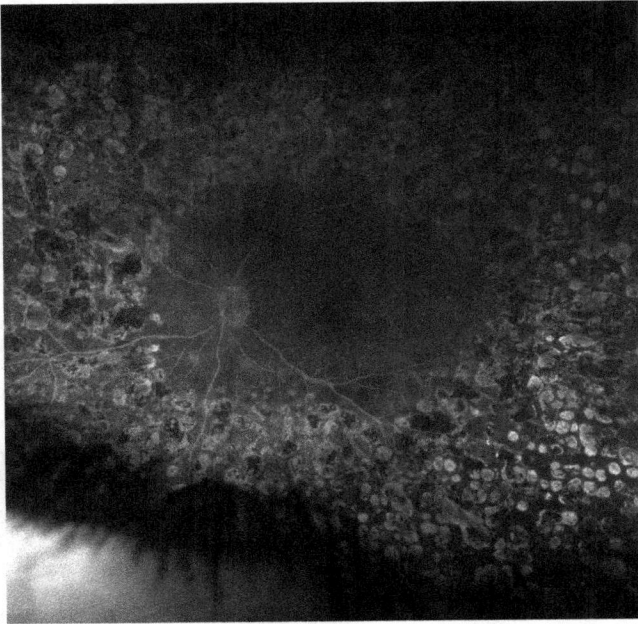

FIGURE 6.6 The ideal posterior border of the traditional PRP laser course.

Patients with NVI can indeed sometimes benefit from an injection of an anti-VEGF agent first to get the disease under control quickly and prevent neovascular glaucoma as much as possible. A single shot of ranibizumab biosimilar followed by a timely course of PRP (completed within 6 weeks) would do the trick. Be wary, though, that just because a patient may be diabetic, any NVI shouldn't automatically be considered to be due to diabetes; if there is no diabetic retinopathy visible, could it be due to say uveitis, retinal detachment or the presence of a tumour? If there is any doubt, then a fundus fluorescein angiography (FFA) can be performed, which will show up any ischaemic retina like a Christmas tree.

On that note, targeted PRP can sometimes be employed if there is a need to preserve as much visual field as possible or if there is some doubt as to the aetiology of the new vessels (an RVO on top of diabetic retinopathy, for instance), whereby the laser would be best targeted in one specific area. Widefield FFA is the usual means to do this; however, with advancing technology, widefield OCT-A is gaining popularity but has not as yet reached the level of reliability or accessibility that would allow dispensing with FFA.

Should PRP be impossible to apply, with a vitreous haemorrhage being the most common reason, then perform a B-scan to rule out any retinal detachment or other such causes (people with diabetes can also get retinal tears and such), then wait 6 weeks to see if it settles enough to apply laser. If, after 6 weeks, the blood still is too thick, then ask your friendly vitreoretinal colleagues for help. If, after 6 weeks, the blood is clearing, but the view is still not good enough, then at a push it might be allowable to wait a further 6 weeks, but if laser is still not possible after this point then the bullet must be bitten and a vitreoretinal referral made for vitrectomy and endolaser.

Christiana Says...

PRP undoubtedly saves vision. However, it is associated with visual field constriction, reduced night vision and reduced contrast sensitivity. Most units in the United Kingdom use multispot laser systems to perform PRP. This method is faster, less painful and causes less collateral damage, which may result in less incidence of PRP-induced macular oedema and visual field constriction. However, the technique described in the Diabetic Retinopathy Study (DRS) and ETDRS study using single-spot argon laser remains the reference standard for treatment of PDR. This is because the evidence for efficacy with the newer multispot laser systems are limited to small studies and, anecdotally, there may be higher rates of persistence of active PDR despite full PRP treatment with these systems. The dream is to have interventions that prevent PDR or treat PDR without destroying the peripheral retina. Such treatments remain elusive.

Now let us discuss treating **diabetic maculopathy**. Anti-VEGF agents are the mainstay of treatment, and it is best to apply them in a treat-and-extend manner with a view to increasing the gap between injections as much as possible, in the same manner as neovascular age-related macular degeneration (nAMD). Should your unit have great capacity, where follow-up injection appointments are not an issue, then cheaper biosimilar anti-VEGF agents can be used such as ranibizumab or Aflibercept 2 mg, but in the real world, where it is common for appointments to slip and capacity is stretched to the breaking point, then longer-acting agents must be used instead. There are two main anti-VEGF agents to consider here: faricimab 6 mg and Aflibercept 8 mg. These are more expensive but last longer and can allow struggling eye units to keep their appointments on time. They should also be considered if the weaker agents either don't allow the injection intervals to be spaced out very far or don't succeed in drying out the retina in the first place.

Treat-and-extend regimes should aim to dry the macula, although DMO is more forgiving and less damaging to the retina and to vision than nAMD by quite some margin. Small amounts of fluid can be tolerated much better. Even still, the best regime is to start with injections every 4 weeks and after drying occurs, extend in either 2-week or 4-week intervals up to 16 weekly injections. Should the patient stay dry even at 16-week injection intervals, then it is reasonable to suspend treatment to see what happens, as with nAMD, with monitoring every 12 weeks or so to ensure the fluid isn't coming back again. Bevacizumab (Avastin) is an alternate anti-VEGF agent but should be recognised as the weakest of the bunch. Should it not cut the mustard, then have a low threshold for converting the patient to a longer-acting, stronger, better agent. Brolicuzumab (Beovu) has been largely abandoned over safety concerns regarding inflammation.

The main difference between nAMD and DMO is that steroid injections can be used with DMO, but have no role whatsoever with nAMD. Dexamethasone injections (Ozurdex) are the main ones used and have additional side effects such as cataract progression and increased intraocular pressure but lack the thromboembolic side effects of anti-VEGF agents. They are stronger than anti-VEGF agents generally, so in phakic patients initially commenced on an anti-VEGF drug should that fail to do anything much after three injections, or five, depending on whether there was some improvement at least after three, then an Ozurdex can be used to try and dry things up. It's a sort of 'nuclear' option that is powerful because it affects inflammatory mediators all across the inflammatory cascade, but also wears off after three to six months and then a decision has to be made whether to re-inject, with each re-injection contributing towards cataract growth. It's also a bit of a bouncy regime with fluid allowed to come back as the capsule dissolves away; there is no such thing as a treat-and-extend Ozurdex regime, but if anti-VEGF agents don't work, there isn't really another option.

In pseudophakic patients, Ozurdex can be considered at an earlier stage, or even from the outset, provided that the patient is not glaucomatous, of course. The main benefit is capacity because after one injection, monitoring is needed around 6 weeks later to check the intraocular pressure and thereafter every 3 months or so to check for fluid returning, whereas with a treat-and-extend regime, there are injection appointments needed every few weeks for a lot longer. Pressure is an issue, but in reality, if one glaucoma drop keeps the pressure under control, then Ozurdex can be repeated and all is well. However, if two agents are required, you're on a bit of a sticky wicket and exposing the patient to danger (and the humiliation of having to ask your glaucoma colleague for help to fix a problem you've caused) and it is best to leave off the steroid in that situation. In short, anti-VEGF in DMO is like a slow and steady infantry attack slowly pushing the front line back with Ozurdex being more akin to a heavy artillery attack with the potential for a major advance but possible collateral damage.

Another longer-acting agent called fluocinolone acetonide (Iluvien) was all the rage a while back as it was billed as being like Ozurdex but lasted 3 years instead of 3 months. It doesn't. If Ozurdex barely controls the oedema, Iluvien stands no chance, but its niche might well be if Ozurdex controls the oedema well, but patients don't want such frequent injections, then Iluvien might be the answer. The hefty price tag is more than a bit off-putting, though.

Now that both laser and injections have been covered, the main bread-and-butter remit of medical retina, the remaining aspects fall into the purview of our vitreoretinal friends. This would include non-resolving vitreous haemorrhages, epiretinal membrane development, tractional retinal detachments or gliotic scarring growth and persistent vitreous haemorrhage despite more than adequate PRP. It is vital to have good relationships with the vitreoretinal team, so such cases can be seen in a timely manner and opinions given and surgery undertaken. If a vitreous haemorrhage does not clear in a timely manner, do not sit on it for months and months and months; send it to the people who can actually do something about it. Lastly, cataract. If a patient has any sort of cataract and is in need of Ozurdex injections, it might be best to bite the bullet and put them on the list rather than wait for a fully developed cataract to occur first.

Christiana Says...

The ETDRS study established laser as the gold standard for clinically significant macular oedema; however, there were associated adverse events with laser. Therefore, the modified ETDRS protocol was developed to simplify treatment and reduce laser-induced retinal damage and is still widely used as an adjunct to anti-VEGF therapy.

Modified ETDRS specification:

Spot size: 50–100 microns
Power: barely visible burn
Spacing: 1 burn-width apart
Pattern: All areas of retinal thickening
Re-treatment: 3–4 months, depending on response
Foveal protection: Avoid the central 500 microns

With regard to a crystal ball to tell us which therapy is best for the patient in front of you, we do not yet have one, despite focused research on various biomarkers. We do, however, have prognostic OCT biomarkers, such as the presence of disorganized retinal inner layers and disruption of the ellipsoid zone, which correlate with visual acuity and their presence at the central subfield can help manage expectations with treatment. Other biomarkers such as hyperreflective foci, diffuse sponge-like macular oedema continue to be investigated for their predictive and prognostic value, and it is likely with the use of AI and big data that we will have the much needed crystal ball soon.

Special Circumstances

Special circumstances include patients with diabetic eye disease undergoing cataract surgery, who are pregnant, who have glaucoma and such. Cataract surgery releases huge quantities of VEGF into the eye and if diabetic retinopathy or maculopathy is uncontrolled, then a sudden and catastrophic deterioration can occur. If there is any new vessel disease present or a touch of rubeosis, cataract surgery can propel the eye into fulminant disease with much haemorrhaging, even during the surgery itself. If a patient needs PRP, do it before surgery, waiting at least 6 weeks afterward for the laser to take effect. If there is macular oedema present in need of treatment, ensure the macula is flat beforehand. Expect surgery to be a fertiliser for deterioration. It is wise to add a non-steroidal agent such as topical Acular tds for 6 weeks after cataract surgery, as well as the usual Maxidex. If trouble is expected, it might even be worth giving a quick shot of biosimilar ranibizumab on the table right after the operation concludes to stave off any trouble. This does have a good effect, of course, but it also makes both patient and surgeon feel better that all precautions have been taken.

Regarding pregnant women, diabetes can quickly and unexpectedly deteriorate, so make sure to keep a close eye on things every 8 to 12 weeks in patients who already have pre-proliferative disease. Laser is fine to apply if needed, but anti-VEGF agents are a big no-no. This is mainly due to a belief that systemic absorption can harm the foetus, though there is no reliable evidence of this in humans. Even still, it is wise to consider leaving any intravitreal treatment until after the birth, if it can wait, or only using Ozurdex if it cannot. Patients with glaucoma should generally avoid steroid implants, and patients with a history of thromboembolic disease should generally avoid anti-VEGF injections if they have had either a myocardial infarction or a cerebrovascular accident within three to 6 months of the time of the proposed injection. Patients expecting to go away for long periods might benefit more from a longer-acting agent. The below flowchart provides a schematic you can follow from diagnosis to management.

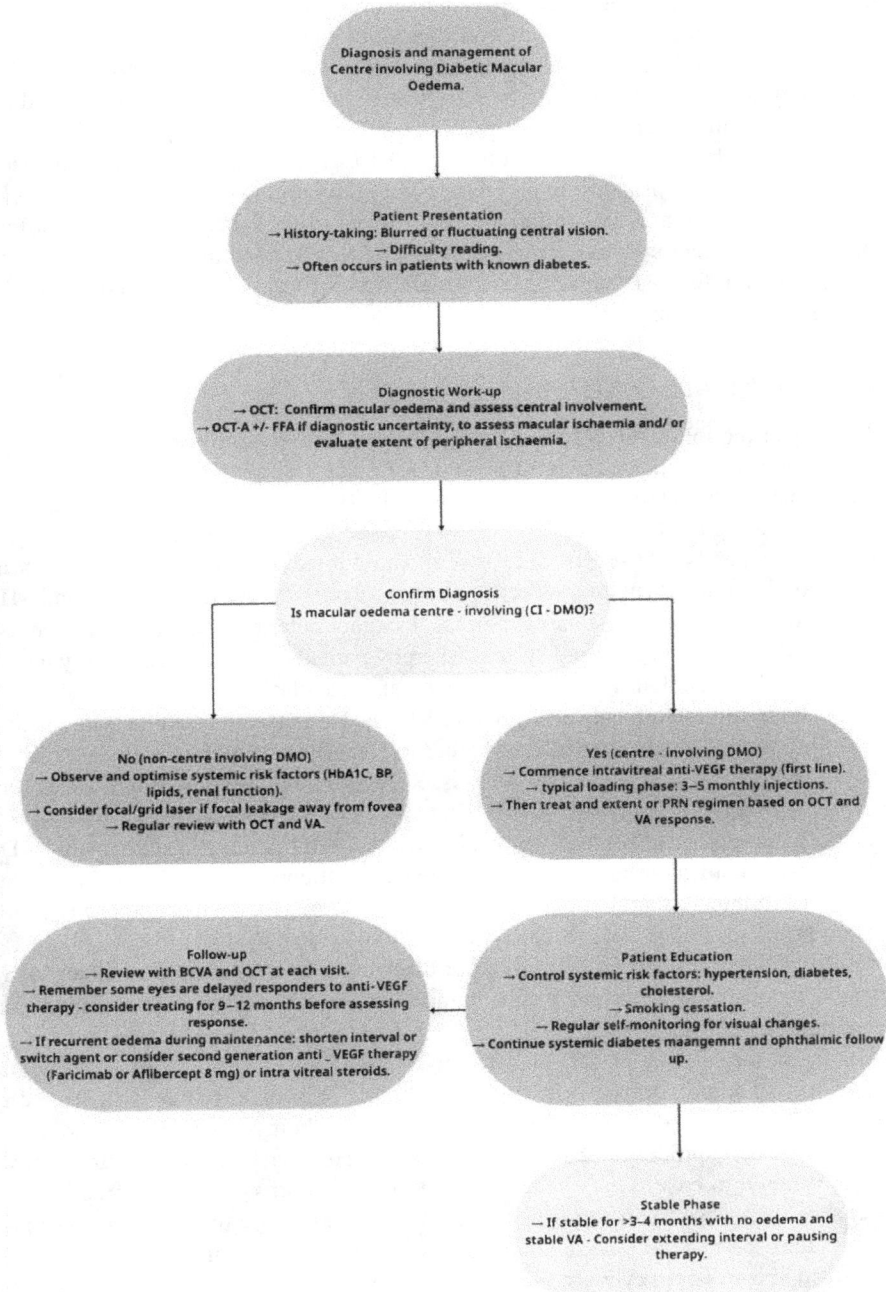

Diagnosis and management of Centre involving Diabetic Macular Oedema.

Patient Presentation
→ History-taking: Blurred or fluctuating central vision.
→ Difficulty reading.
→ Often occurs in patients with known diabetes.

Diagnostic Work-up
→ OCT: Confirm macular oedema and assess central involvement.
→ OCT-A +/- FFA if diagnostic uncertainty, to assess macular ischaemia and/ or evaluate extent of peripheral ischaemia.

Confirm Diagnosis
Is macular oedema centre - involving (CI - DMO)?

No (non-centre involving DMO)
→ Observe and optimise systemic risk factors (HbA1C, BP, lipids, renal function).
→ Consider focal/grid laser if focal leakage away from fovea
→ Regular review with OCT and VA.

Yes (centre - involving DMO)
→ Commence intravitreal anti-VEGF therapy (first line).
→ typical loading phase: 3–5 monthly injections.
→ Then treat and extent or PRN regimen based on OCT and VA response.

Follow-up
→ Review with BCVA and OCT at each visit.
→ Remember some eyes are delayed responders to anti-VEGF therapy - consider treating for 9–12 months before assessing response.
→ If recurrent oedema during maintenance: shorten interval or switch agent or consider second generation anti _ VEGF therapy (Faricimab or Aflibercept 8 mg) or intra vitreal steroids.

Patient Education
→ Control systemic risk factors: hypertension, diabetes, cholesterol.
→ Smoking cessation.
→ Regular self-monitoring for visual changes.
→ Continue systemic diabetes maangemnt and ophthalmic follow up.

Stable Phase
→ If stable for >3–4 months with no oedema and stable VA - Consider extending interval or pausing therapy.

Christiana Says...

Concerns about intravitreal anti-VEGF in pregnancy centre on the central role of VEGF in the maintenance of fetal and placental vasculature. However, there is no data from controlled studies because pregnant women are systematically excluded. Case series abound, but findings are confounded by the high background rate of mis-carriages and inherently high-risk pregnancies in women with pre-existing diabetes. There may well be circumstances where intravitreal therapy must be considered in a pregnant woman (for example, a pregnant woman with bilateral high-risk PDR that continues to progress despite bilateral PRP). Again, there is insufficient data on which anti-VEGF is safest in pregnancy, but ranibizumab is most often used as it has the lowest systemic absorption and shortest half-life. Where possible, avoiding anti-VEGF therapy in the first trimester is advisable, given the inherently higher risk of teratogenic effects at that stage. Above all, these patients should be co-managed with their obstetrician.

FOLLOW-UP ALGORITHMS

The simpler the follow-up plan and the flow of patients through and around the diabetic eye service is, the easier it is for everyone – doctors, non-medical practitioners and patients – to understand and follow. Simplicity is key. The number of patients actually needing treatment is the tip of the diabetic iceberg, and seeing every single one of the patients referred from DESW (or an equivalent screening service) in a consultant-led clinic is neither effective nor practical. Far better to filter R2 and M1 patients (eye screening systems without OCT cannot determine whether a patient is M1A or M1S) through a virtual system whereby patients receive visual acuity tests, dilation, widefield colour fundus photography and macular OCT scan. These images can be taken by technicians and reviewed by non-medical practitioners in medical retina, who can then determine whether to send them to a consultant-led clinic. Patients with suspected active new vessels, R3A, should be seen within 2 weeks (or 4 at most) in a laser clinic to apply the first shots of PRP. As a general guide, M1A and R2 patients should be seen within 12 weeks. DMO is *not* the same as nAMD and the 2-week macular target does not apply here. Patients can be followed up twice in a virtual clinic system, but every third visit should be face-to-face; otherwise, the system promotes alienation and apathy amongst patients and staff alike.

R3S patients can be seen every year, or discharged to screening if possible; M1S every 6 months and R2 every 3 to 6 months. Make full use of your non-medical practitioners (see Chapter 11).

In the United kingdom, the Diabetic Eye Screening Programme (DESP) is an incredible standard and now incorporates OCT. This means that patients with resolved DMO can be confidently discharged to c if their retinopathy is also non-referrable with confidence that they will be referred back if they recur. In my clinic, we tend to ensure they have had at least 6–9 months recurrence-free before discharge. It is wise to ensure eyes treated for PDR are truly quiescent before discharge; fibrosed neovascularisation, venous calibre close to normal, well-lasered as described above. These eyes are therefore at low risk of recurrence and can be safely monitored once a year.

WHAT IS THE FUTURE FOR DIABETIC RETINOPATHY AND DMO?

The interventions in late-stage development are focused on reducing the burden of treatment through surgical implants requiring refills once in 6 or 9 months; by topical delivery, which the patient performs 3–6 times a day at home at their convenience; or through gene therapy (one and done!). For diabetic retinopathy, fenofibrate may help slow progression, surgical implants are also an option here, as is gene therapy. Underlying diabetic retinopathy is the systemic disease, and strong evidence that optimizing glycemic control significantly reduces the risk of diabetic retinopathy progression. The introduction of GLP-1 Receptor agonists and SGLT2 inhibitors, in addition to hybrid closed-loop systems, which have all been shown to result in significant optimization of glycemic control, may ultimately play the most transformative role in reducing the risk of diabetic retinopathy progression.

REFERENCES

1. Rai BB, Maddess T, Nolan CJ. Functional diabetic retinopathy: A new concept to improve management of diabetic retinal diseases. Surv Ophthalmol. 2025; 70(2):232–240. doi: 10.1016/j.survophthal.2024.11.010. Epub 2024 Nov 23.
2. Lawrenson JG, Bourmpaki E, Bunce C, Stratton IM, Gardner P, Anderson J; EROS Study Group. Trends in diabetic retinopathy screening attendance and associations with vision impairment attributable to diabetes in a large nationwide cohort. Diabet Med. 2021; 38(4):e14425. doi: 10.1111/dme.14425. Epub 2020 Nov 1.
3. Early Treatment Diabetic Retinopathy Study Research Group. Early photocoagulation for diabetic retinopathy. ETDRS report number 9. Ophthalmology. 1991; 98(5 Suppl):766–785.
4. Writing Committee for the Diabetic Retinopathy Clinical Research Network. Panretinal photocoagulation vs intravitreous ranibizumab for proliferative diabetic retinopathy: A randomized clinical trial. JAMA. 2015; 314:2137–2146.
5. Sivaprasad S, Prevost AT, Vasconcelos JC, Riddell A, Murphy C, Kelly J, Bainbridge J, Tudor-Edwards R, Hopkins D, Hykin P; CLARITY Study Group. Clinical efficacy of intravitreal aflibercept versus panretinal photocoagulation for best corrected visual acuity in patients with proliferative diabetic retinopathy at 52 weeks (CLARITY): A multicentre, single-blinded, randomised, controlled, phase 2b, non-inferiority trial. Lancet. 2017; 389(10085):2193–2203. doi: 10.1016/S0140-6736(17)31193-5. Epub 2017 May 7.
6. Wykoff CC, Eichenbaum DA, Roth DB, Hill L, Fung AE, Haskova Z. Ranibizumab induces regression of diabetic retinopathy in most patients at high risk of progression to proliferative diabetic retinopathy. Ophthalmol Retina. 2018; 2(10):997–1009. doi: 10.1016/j.oret.2018.06.005. Epub 2018 Aug 1.
7. Keech AC et al. Effect of fenofibrate on the need for laser treatment for diabetic retinopathy (FIELD study): A randomised controlled trial. Lancet. 2007; 370(9600):1687–1697.
8. ACCORD Study Group and ACCORD Eye Study Group. Effects of medical therapies on retinopathy progression in type 2 diabetes. N Engl J Med. 2010; 363(3):233–244.
9. Preiss D, Logue J, Sammons E, Zayed M, Emberson J, Wade R, Wallendszus K, Stevens W, Cretney R, Harding S, Leese G, Currie G, Armitage J. Effect of fenofibrate on progression of diabetic retinopathy. NEJM Evid. 2024; 3(8):EVIDoa2400179. doi: 10.1056/EVIDoa2400179. Epub 2024 Jun 21.
10. Early Treatment Diabetic Retinopathy Study Research Group. Photocoagulation for diabetic macular edema. Early treatment diabetic retinopathy study report number 1. Arch Ophthalmol. 1985; 103(12):1796–1806.

11. Nguyen QD, Brown DM, Marcus DM et al. Ranibizumab for diabetic macular edema: Results from 2 phase III randomized trials: RISE and RIDE. Ophthalmology. 2012; 119(4):789–801.
12. Korobelnik JF, Do DV, Schmidt-Erfurth U et al. Intravitreal aflibercept for diabetic macular edema. Ophthalmology. 2014; 121(6):2247–2254.
13. Wells JA, Glassman AR; Diabetic Retinopathy Clinical Research Network et al. Aflibercept, bevacizumab, or ranibizumab for diabetic macular edema. N Engl J Med. 2015; 372(13):1193–1203.
14. Augustin AJ, Kuppermann BD, Lanzetta P, Loewenstein A, Li XY, Cui H, Hashad Y, Whitcup SM; Ozurdex MEAD Study Group. Dexamethasone intravitreal implant in previously treated patients with diabetic macular edema: Subgroup analysis of the MEAD study. BMC Ophthalmol. 2015; 15:150. doi: 10.1186/s12886-015-0148-2.
15. Campochiaro PA, Brown DM, Pearson A et al. Sustained delivery fluocinolone acetonide vitreous inserts provide benefit for at least 3 years in patients with diabetic macular edema. Ophthalmology. 2012; 119:2125–2132. doi: 10.1016/j.ophtha.2012.04.030.
16. Wykoff CC, Abreu F, Adamis AP, Basu K, Eichenbaum DA, Haskova Z, Lin H, Loewenstein A, Mohan S, Pearce IA, Sakamoto T, Schlottmann PG, Silverman D, Sun JK, Wells JA, Willis JR, Tadayoni R; YOSEMITE and RHINE Investigators. Efficacy, durability, and safety of intravitreal faricimab with extended dosing up to every 16 weeks in patients with diabetic macular oedema (YOSEMITE and RHINE): Two randomised, double-masked, phase 3 trials. Lancet. 2022; 399(10326):741–755. doi: 10.1016/S0140-6736(22)00018-6. Epub 2022 Jan 24.
17. Brown DM, Boyer DS, Do DV, Wykoff CC, Sakamoto T, Win P, Joshi S, Salehi-Had H, Seres A, Berliner AJ, Leal S, Vitti R, Chu KW, Reed K, Rao R, Cheng Y, Sun W, Voronca D, Bhore R, Schmidt-Ott U, Schmelter T, Schulze A, Zhang X, Hirshberg B, Yancopoulos GD, Sivaprasad S; PHOTON Investigators. Intravitreal aflibercept 8 mg in diabetic macular oedema (PHOTON): 48-week results from a randomised, double-masked, non-inferiority, phase 2/3 trial. Lancet. 2024; 403(10432):1153–1163. doi: 10.1016/S0140-6736(23)02577-1. Epub 2024 Mar 7.
18. Writing Committee for the Diabetic Retinopathy Clinical Research Network (DRCR. net). Comparison of the modified early treatment diabetic retinopathy study and mild macular grid laser photocoagulation strategies for diabetic macular edema. Arch Ophthalmol. 2007; 125(4):469–480.

7 Retinal Vein Occlusions

The little brother in the triplet 'big three' of medical retina, neovascular age-related macular degeneration (nAMD), diabetic eye disease and retinal vein occlusion (RVO), vein occlusions may well be fewer in number but are equally blinding should they occur with their pathophysiology and treatment being remarkably similar to diabetes. Indeed, as discussed in Chapter 6, diabetes is one of many factors that can contribute to RVO, and looking for undiagnosed diabetes is part of the workup. The good news is that prognosis-wise, although diabetes is a chronic condition, RVO has a peak impact that usually improves spontaneously over time on a spectrum from total and complete resolution to residual chronic disease not as bad as the peak but perhaps not far off it. In a way, due to the potential self-limiting nature of the condition, treatment can be regarded as nursing the eye through the worst of it so that as much vision as possible is preserved by the end of the illness. College guidance mandates that patients with RVO are seen and treated within 6 weeks of referral.

Systematic review informs us that the natural history of macula oedema secondary to branch RVO (BRVO) can be one of improvement, with mean visual acuity improving by up to three lines over 18 months. However, many of these eyes remain below driving vision. For example, the BVOS reported spontaneous resolution in 34% of eyes to 0.30 LogMAR or better by year 3. Eyes with central retinal vein occlusion (CRVO) often have a more severe course, unless they are non-ischaemic, in which case any associated macular oedema resolves in about one-third of eyes with retinal neovascularisation occurring very infrequently. We must remember that long-term unresolved macular oedema results in irreversible sight loss and ischaemic changes drive retinal neovascularisation, which in severe cases can culminate in rubeotic glaucoma, an outcome to avoid at all costs. Advances in imaging and therapeutics over the past three decades have thankfully reduced the incidence of irreversible sight loss due to RVO.

CAUSES

Nothing comes from nothing, as the saying goes; everything has a cause. The frustrating thing with RVO is that more often than not, no cause is detected. Important associations include hypertension, diabetes, systemic inflammatory conditions and multiple haematological conditions that affect the viscosity of the blood, though there are countless others. If a patient presents with a typical vein occlusion and is a typical looking patient over the age of, say, 60 years, then performing only the tests recommended by the Royal College of Ophthalmologists (RCOphth) is the best thing. Don't go fishing for everything under the sun because you will indeed find red herrings everywhere. What will you do with a peculiar thyroid function test or liver result that has nothing to do with why the RVO happened in the first place? Refer to

DOI: 10.1201/9781003628309-7

another specialty with a letter that will surely frustrate and cause all sorts of problems? Or keep quiet about the result until something happens down the line and the patient then asks why nothing was done by the clinician ordering the test, the hapless ophthalmologist, although the condition in question has nothing to do with why the patient presented.

The RCOphth recommends blood pressure measurement, a full blood count (FBC), erythrocyte sedimentation rate (ESR) and glucose as standard tests with the option of adding others as the situation demands. Blood pressure should be done in clinic because it is not too infrequently that exotic levels of pressure are found, though anything higher than 160 systolic and 90 diastolic are significant. Any high reading less than 200 systolic or 100 diastolic can be sent to the general practitioner (GP) for urgent attention because hospital medical teams tend to become hostile to ophthalmologists referring random high blood pressures in asymptomatic (from a blood pressure perspective, headache and such) patients, while they are busy saving lives in overstretched teams. It is also unwise for a humble eye doctor who last did 'proper' medicine decades ago to go prescribing what they consider appropriate antihypertensive agents; leave it to the experts, leave it to the people who will have to monitor things going forward.

If the blood pressure is indeed over 200 systolic or 100 diastolic, or both, then unfortunately the bullet must be bitten, and a phone call made to the medical registrar on call to refer the patient. At these levels, there is genuine danger to life and a haemorrhagic cerebrovascular accident can be prevented by timely referral. Obviously, this isn't a hard cutoff level, that would be ludicrous, and other factors such as symptoms of headache or general debility need to be taken into account in deciding to refer there and then. The authors have seen cases of patients presenting with an RVO where no blood pressure was taken, and between the presenting appointment and the follow-up, the patient was admitted with malignant hypertension after having suffered a devastating event of some sort. Measuring the blood pressure in clinic is sacrosanct. It is not worth asking the patient to 'get it checked with their GP practice' because it is so monstrously difficult to get an appointment in this climate that you might as well be asking the patient to phone the president of the United States to ask for world peace. Some practices are, of course, very good, though.

An FBC looks for any strange blood conditions (there is a long list) that can make the blood coagulate more readily. There is no purpose in asking for more detailed haematological tests unless some condition is suspected. Plus, normal ophthalmologists don't know a huge amount about this and can cause our haematology colleagues annoyance with letters and referrals. Conditions include things such as Waldenstrom macroglobulinaemia and protein c and s deficiency, for instance. Do you remember the coagulation cascade? We thought not. A blood glucose can be used to look for diabetes if there is no diabetes ostensibly present, though a HbA1c is arguably better. An ESR is good as a blanket test to look for inflammatory conditions generally.

Any other tests should be done in an otherwise 'typical' patient, depending on symptoms. For example, if you suspect sarcoidosis, you could ask for an angiotensin-converting enzyme (ACE); if you suspect antiphospholipid syndrome, you could ask for an anticardiolipin antibody and so on. But less is more. If, however, a patient is unusual in some way, say the person is young or has other associated ophthalmic or systemic features, then instead of the usual general history, a more detailed focused history needs to be taken. Ophthalmic history might include angle closure glaucoma or surgery, while systemic history might include inherited conditions or inflammatory diseases.

The base mechanism is that the vein becomes blocked, and it is thought that the surrounding adventitial layer that binds the vein to the artery in the retina contributes to this situation because an expanded artery compresses a vein and a compressed vein alters the blood flow (remember Virchow's Triad?) and can cause it to block. Arteriovenous nipping, 'A-V nipping', is the body's sign that this compression is taking place in a hypertensive patient. The vein can become blocked in the optic nerve, causing the whole retina or one of the branches to be affected. Perhaps some sort of congenital design flaw in one place, or many, creates a weak spot, a pinchable location. This can result in trouble if the blood pressure goes up, or if the blood pressure goes up to a lesser extent in the context of other predisposing factors, or with those predisposing factors alone with a normal blood pressure.

Christiana Says...

The pathogenesis of RVO is multifactorial, involving a combination of vascular, anatomic, and biochemical mediators associated with systemic diseases that result in occlusion or thrombus formation. The most commonly accepted mechanism for branch RVO is compression of the retinal vein by an overlying sclerotic artery at an arteriovenous crossing. This shared adventitial sheath predisposes the vein to compression, turbulent flow and thrombus formation. Atherosclerosis in the retinal arteries is a key contributing factor to this compressive pathology (1). Hypertension, diabetes mellitus and hyperlipidemia are strongly associated with BRVO, likely due to the associated vascular endothelial dysfunction and arteriosclerosis.

Traditionally, CRVO was also thought of as a thrombotic disorder, with the central retinal vein and central retinal artery sharing a common adventitial sheath at the level of the lamina cribrosa in the optic nerve head. The vein is compressed by the adjacent sclerotic artery, leading to turbulent blood flow, endothelial damage and thrombus formation (2). More recently, CRVO is no longer viewed as a simple thrombotic disorder, with alteration of blood flow velocity and impaired vessel integrity now also considered important to its occurrence. Even fundamental facts, such as the site of occlusion in CRVO, are disputed, with some believing it occurs at the lamina cribrosa and others suggesting it occurs posterior to this. This is not totally unimportant as the site of occlusion influences whether, albeit rare, potential therapeutic interventions can be carried out, such as in the past when surgical decompression of the central retinal vein was undertaken if the blockage was at the lamina cribrosa (3).

Special consideration is made for RVO occurring in younger patients (typically less than 50 years old) and in patients presenting with bilateral RVO. In this group, a prothrombotic or inflammatory causes may be implicated, although in some cases, no underlying cause is identified. Table 7.1 illustrates potential causes of atypical RVO.

TABLE 7.1

Atypical Causes of RVO

Conditions to Consider in Atypical RVO	Example
Thrombophilia	Factor V Leiden, Protein V/S deficiency, hyperhomocysteinaemia
Autoimmune/inflammatory	APS, SLE, Behcet
Hormonal	Oral contraceptives/HRT
Mechanical/ocular	Glaucoma/Optic disc drusen
Infectious	Syphilis/TB

DIAGNOSIS

While the cause of RVO is of course important, diagnosing the RVO itself as an RVO is what comes first. In reality, patients are usually diagnosed by optometrists outside the hospital or colleagues in another subspecialty within, and the letter itself mentions 'vein occlusion' in some way. Patients also have an optical coherence tomography (OCT) scan performed in clinic (and occasionally a widefield image), and before we have even uttered one word to them or seen their face, we know almost always what the diagnosis is because we have kind of cheated, we have been forewarned. Hence the reason the 'cases' section was placed above, though it does sort of seem like putting the cart before the horse.

Vein occlusions come in a variety of forms; a CRVO, where the whole retina is involved, a hemiretinal vein occlusion (HRVO), where either the superior or inferior half of the retina is affected, and a BRVO, where anything from a quadrant of retina is involved down to a small macular branch vein occlusion that can mimic nAMD. The hallmarks are flame haemorrhages because it is the retinal venous vasculature that is affected, and these run in the innermost, most superficial layers of the retina and the blood, and therefore tends to orient itself along the nerve fibre layer direction. There can also be other signs of ischaemia, including anything seen in diabetic eye disease: cotton wool spots, hard exudates and new vessels, for example. New vessels can occur at the disc (NVD), the iris (NVI), or elsewhere (NVE) as with diabetes; again, with a propensity for neovascular glaucoma to develop. In fact, so-called 100-day glaucoma, which sounds like a fitness challenge, is so named because it takes approximately 100 days (though also potentially a lot longer) for an RVO to lead to pressure increases following peripheral anterior synechiae developing as a result of NVI.

There is a spectrum, of course, depending on the degree of blockage, and therefore the amount of vascular endothelial growth factor (VEGF) released into the eye. The quickest estimate for neovascular glaucoma development is indeed 100 days, when usually a catastrophic sort of blockage has occurred full of ischaemia and blood, and the eye is flooded with VEGF; zero to 60 in 100 days. Lesser amounts of ischaemia have lesser amounts of VEGF release, lesser signs and symptoms and lesser chance of neovascularisation. Interestingly, BRVOs and HRVOs especially are most likely to cause neovascularisation, more so than CRVOs, with macular BRVOs

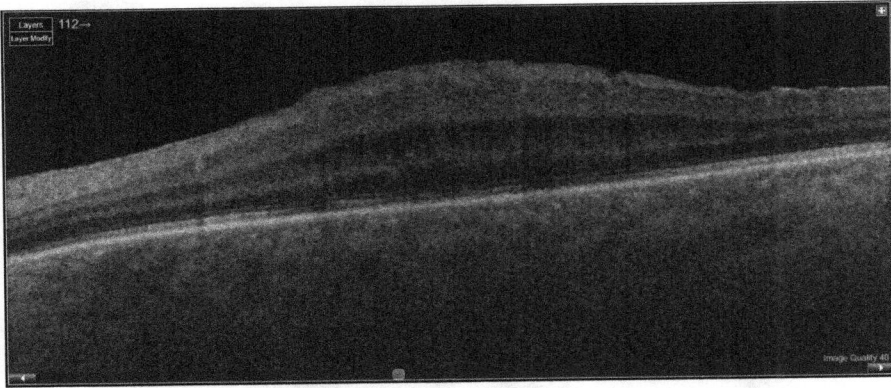

FIGURE 7.1 Optical coherence tomography (OCT) scan of a patient with macular branch retinal vein occlusion (BRVO).

rarely (nothing is ever 'never' in medicine) releasing enough VEGF to cause issues. It is much more complex an inflammatory milieu than VEGF alone, and involves a whole host of inflammatory mediators, which is why intravitreal dexamethasone in the form of Ozurdex does so well. Nevertheless, the reason HRVOs do worse than CRVOs neovascularisation-wise might be due to the fact that there is some tissue left alive to call for help and become inflamed. As Machiavelli states in *The Prince*, 'if an injury has to be done to a man it must be so severe that his vengeance need not be feared;' applied to the retina then, if the injury done by the RVO is so severe that it kills the retina, then it is better in a way than if it only half kills the retina. Dead men can't call for help, where VEGF is the call and neovascular disease is the help.

Differentiating between other causes of the fundal appearance usually means differentiating between RVO and either diabetes or nAMD. Obviously, only macular BRVOs can be confused with nAMD, but clues lie in the distribution of fluid disproportionately on one side or the other of the horizontal midline of the eye and normal retinal pigment epithelium (RPE) on OCT scanning. Figure 7.1 displays an OCT scan of an eye with macular branch vein occlusion; note the intact RPE and thickness contour lines displaying predominantly one-sided fluid.

Diabetes can indeed be mistaken for a mild CRVO, as there are scanty haemorrhages in all four quadrants. However, a severe CRVO with a so-called stormy sunset appearance of deep haemorrhages, such that there is much more blood than there is seen in a regular CRVO, and should never be mistaken for diabetes. The stormy sunset descriptor is meant to make the ophthalmologist think of a sun setting in a red, angry, cloud-filled sky, where the disc represents the sun and the bloody fundus the surrounding red cloudy swirls. Figure 7.2 illustrates the appearance of a stormy sunset CRVO. The more flame shaped the haemorrhage, the more superficial they are and the more likely it is going to be due to a vein occlusion as a result. Dual pathology can be tricky, however.

Other differential diagnoses include hypertensive retinopathy, which is one of the reasons (the other is that hypertension can directly cause an RVO to occur) it is so

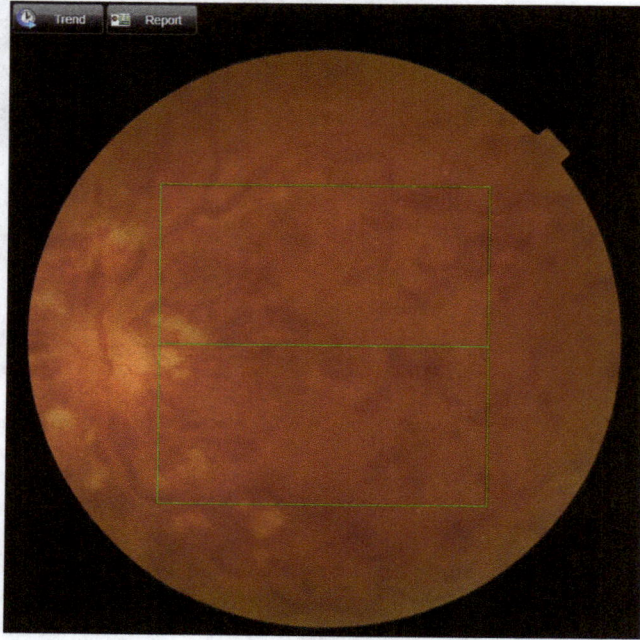

FIGURE 7.2 'Stormy sunset' of a severe central retinal vein occlusion (CRVO).

important to measure blood pressure in all new patients. Most of the time, though, an RVO presents as a unilateral disease, whilst diabetes and hypertensive retinopathy usually have signs in both eyes. Signs can be asymmetric, however, particularly in patients with ocular ischaemic syndrome (OIS). The last differential of note is radiation retinopathy, although this is almost always in the context of a choroidal melanoma that has been treated with radiotherapy. However, it is worth bearing in mind if you are referred a patient with a history of choroidal melanoma who now has an apparent vein occlusion in the same eye. There is a long list of other differential diagnoses that are stated to potentially mimic an RVO, but these are the only ones that matter (see Table 7.2).

TABLE 7.2
Differential Diagnosis and Features of Various Causes of Retinal Haemorrhage

Feature	CRVO	OIS	DR
Onset	Sudden	Gradual	Gradual
Laterality	Often unilateral	Unilateral	Bilateral
Vein calibre	Dilated and tortuous	Dilated	Mildly dilated
Haemorrhage distribution	4 quadrants	Mid-peripheral	Mild to severe depending on stage
Cotton-wool spots	Often present	May be present	Can be present
Systemic association	Vascular risk factors	Carotid stenosis	Diabetes mellitus

GRADING SEVERITY

A handy grading system exists with diabetic eye disease to help grade the severity, but no such system exists for RVO. Instead, an unhelpful 'ischaemic versus non-ischaemic' binary classification is used. In reality, there is a spectrum of severity ranging from barely perceptible to hugely, massively, totally ischaemic with no distinct cutoff. There have been attempts to create some sort of limit for defining when an eye with an RVO becomes ischaemic, either by clinical features or fundus fluorescein angiography (FFA) appearance, but this is largely academic for the regular coal face clinician. Far better to simply remember that the worse it looks, the more ischaemic it is likely to be, though widefield FFA and newer technologies such as widefield OCT angiography (OCT-A) can make some sort of estimate of how much retina is not being perfused properly. You could argue that this is not useful; however, as treatment for new vessels is the same regardless – retinal laser – though you could also argue that an attempt to tailor panretinal photocoagulation (PRP) specifically to only the ischaemic areas is in the patient's best interest (see below).

Things to watch for include a relative afferent pupillary defect (RAPD; make sure to ask the nursing staff to look for this prior to dilation), visual acuity, degree of haemorrhage, the presence of disc swelling and just general badness. The worse it looks, the more likely the eye is to become neovascular, and prognosis and advice can be tailored accordingly for the patient. It might not seem like much, but when nothing useful can be done other than looking out for ischaemia, patients appreciate very much an honest prognosis over false optimism.

Regarding the maculopathy side of things, the main distinction is with fluid that will likely respond to treatment and fluid that it is utterly purposeless to try to treat. In this regard, it is similar to diabetic macular oedema (DMO; see Chapter 6). It is a slight catch-22 situation; in fact, as fluid on OCT that is acute, symmetrical, with nice, ordered cysts and a nice profile mirroring Tryfan, the Eiger or some other triangular mountain will almost certainly respond well to treatment because the essential architecture of the retina is preserved (see Figure 7.3). However, on the other hand,

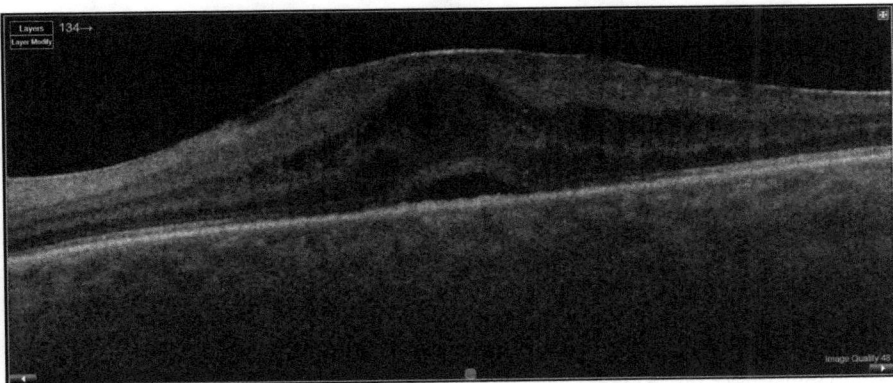

FIGURE 7.3   An OCT profile of cystoid macular oedema secondary to RVO that is likely to respond well to treatment.

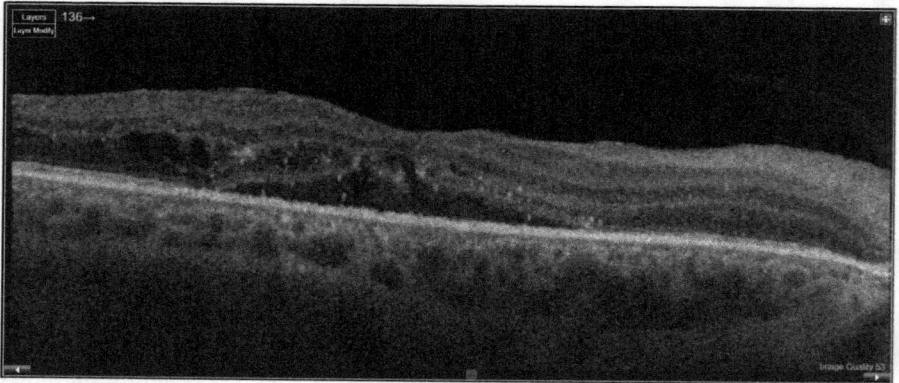

FIGURE 7.4 An OCT profile of cystoid macular oedema secondary to RVO that is unlikely to respond well to treatment.

this is also the sort of fluid that is most likely to resolve spontaneously given time. Chronic fluid that is irregular, spread out over a wider area, has very large spaces within it and resembles a profile of Fan Hir, Crib Goch or some other shallower ridge-like mountain, is unlikely to respond well to treatment because the architecture of the retina has been degraded and abused, and you tend to have an innate sense that treatment wouldn't do very much of anything (see Figure 7.4). The aim of treatment at the end of the day is not to make the retina look more normal, but to alleviate the patient's symptoms or prognosis in some way.

Again, there is no distinct cutoff, and it is a sliding scale between one type and another. Whilst it is fair to say that an OCT-A would be very good at assessing the degree of macular ischaemia present and therefore the likely response (or lack of) to treatment, the reality is that sometimes even ischaemic maculae seem to respond well to treatment, though oftentimes do not, and hence it is often worth giving injections a shot depending on the situation. Perhaps one day we will live in an artificial intelligence (AI) age where investigations will determine not only how successful treatment might be but whether to treat, but this is a long way off and ultimately, the better the AI system is likely to be, the more likely it will be as well that it would not necessarily have human interests as a top priority in its semi-sentient mind. So until then, although there are efforts to grade severity, this is less clinically useful an endeavour than at first it might appear.

Lastly, a good sign – collaterals. These can be either at the disc or in the retina and can at first glance give the appearance of new vessels because they are abnormally dilated and curl in an abnormally tortuous manner, but they are not directionless or purposeless. They are bypass mechanisms where blood is shunted from an overloaded section of venous infrastructure via a usually quiet route to a lower-pressure section beyond the blockage, resulting in a dilated twisty appearance. If Fabian Way, the main route in and out of Swansea, was reduced to only one lane of traffic by, say, roadworks at the Amazon warehouse, then traffic would flow in much greater amounts than usual up Pentreguinea Road, and snaking traffic would be seen by helicopter view twisting up the valley as cars try to reach the M4 at Junction 44 instead of the usual 42. It is a sign that the body is trying to adapt, and with time, the other

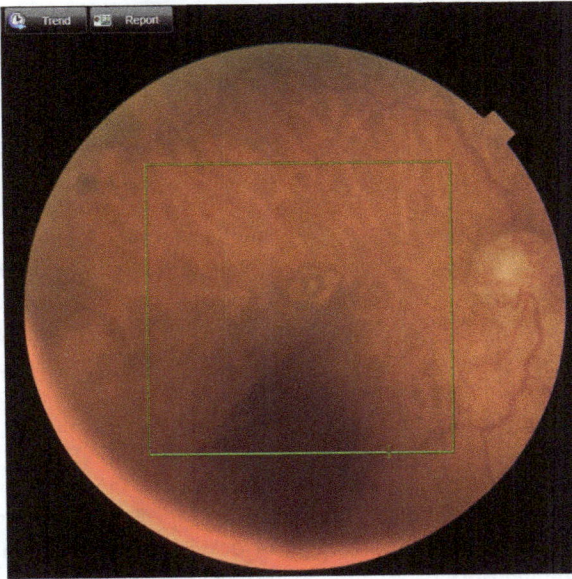

FIGURE 7.5   Disc collaterals.

routes can expand to carry more traffic. Figure 7.5 shows disc collaterals, and Figure 7.6 displays intraretinal collaterals.

Without collateral development, the gridlock situation in Swansea (or indeed any city) would stagnate and worsen, and there is even a chance that as the entire city centre gets bogged up, traffic cannot even make it into the city due to the pressure of cars. Similarly, the very worst CRVOs can actually lead to arterial occlusions, such is the level of venous pressure.

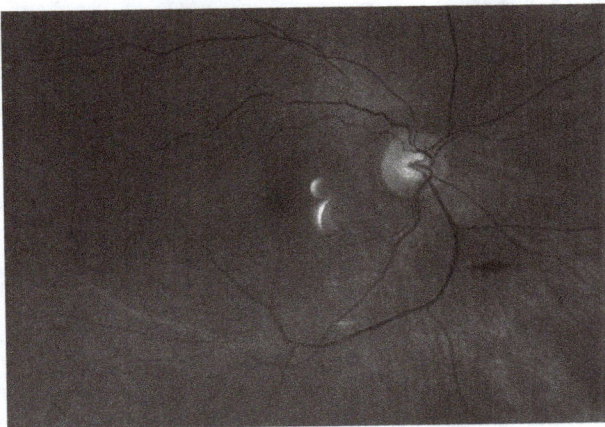

FIGURE 7.6   Intraretinal collaterals.

Christiana Says...

The classification of RVO into ischaemic and non-ischaemic types still influences frequency of monitoring, management and prognostication. Robust evidence from natural history studies and systematic reviews tells us that the visual outcome is different between these two subtypes. For CRVO, ischaemic eyes were defined as those with 10 or more disc areas of capillary non-perfusion (NP), whilst for BRVO, ischaemic eyes were defined as those with 5 or more disc areas of capillary NP. These landmark studies used colour fundus photographs and fluorescein angiographic images using 30- to 60-degree-angle cameras with conventional 7–8 fields covering the posterior pole and mid-periphery.

In recent times, ultra-widefield fluorescein angiography (UWFA) has increasingly replaced conventional FFA due to the ability to capture over 200 degrees of retina compared to 80 degrees with conventional imaging. Findings from studies using UWFA suggest it can be used to better predict the risk of neovascularisation. Nicholson et al. reported 0% of eyes with neovascularisation in eyes with <10 disc areas (DAs) of NP, 14.3% of eyes in eyes with 10–30 DAs of NP, 20% of eyes in eyes with 30–75 DAs of NP and 80% risk in eyes with 75–150 DAs of NP. It also appears that the distribution of ischaemia is important, with posterior pole ischaemia being associated with a significantly higher risk of developing neovascularisation, independent of the amount of ischaemia in the periphery (4).

The Central Vein Occlusion Study (CVOS) still informs many aspects of management today. At the time of the study, clinicians were convinced from clinical experience that eyes with NVI or new vessels at the angle (NVA) needed treatment immediately and were happy to monitor eyes with no significant ischaemia. However, at that time, there was equipoise about whether to treat eyes with significant ischaemia but no NVI or NVA. In addition, the benefits of macular grid laser for macular oedema complicating CRVO were not clear.

This study proved that eyes with significant haemorrhage preventing diagnosis of capillary NP with fluorescein angiography were designated as 'indeterminate' and monitored monthly. Of those eyes, 83% became ischaemic within 4 months, signifying the importance of severe haemorrhagic CRVO as a sign of significant ischaemia and need for close monitoring (5).

In the CVOS trial, three risk factors for progression to ischaemic from non-ischaemic were identified: 5–9 DAs of NP at baseline, visual acuity less than 20/200, and duration of CRVO of less than 1 month. These findings still inform our management of newly presenting CRVO today, with careful monitoring for 4 to 6 weeks for the first 3–4 months to capture eyes that convert to ischaemic CRVO and manage appropriately. The continued use of ultra-widefield fundus photography (UWF-FP) and UWF-FFA will refine our risk-stratification and better inform which eyes we treat prophylactically with laser and which we leave alone.

MANAGEMENT

There are several different aspects of managing a patient with RVO; finding the cause (if any), treating neovascularisation and treating macular oedema. We have addressed finding the cause above, so let us now address the other two aspects. Most importantly, as stated above, patients should be seen and treated (if needed) within 6 weeks of referral according to RCOphth guidelines.

RETINAL ISCHAEMIA AND NEOVASCULARISATION

If a patient presents with any RVO short of a macular BRVO, then watching for neo-vascularisation is the most important thing. If after checking for NVDs or NVEs in the fundus none are seen, always remember to look for NVIs, especially the angle. If there is widespread ischaemic change towards the severe side of the spectrum, then it is imperative to look closely, especially at the iris. If fundal new vessels are found in the context of a highly ischaemic CRVO, then it would be wise to plan a course of immediate PRP laser exactly as you would in a diabetic patient. Should new vessels be found at the iris and/or angle, then there is controversy regarding when and how an injection of anti-VEGF agent should be used. Grey areas are bad for decision-making, so it is sensible to give an injection of biosimilar ranibizumab (or equiva-lent) right away so that in the time it takes laser to be performed (which should be started within 2 weeks) and to take effect, you will have reduced the chances of anterior peripheral synechiae development and intractable neovascular glaucoma. The harm done by not giving an injection is almost always going to be higher than the harm of giving one.

There is no real purpose in performing an FFA to target treatment in a heavily ischaemic eye with neovascularisation because the more, the better, and it is better not to spare the horses. With HRVOs and BRVOs (proper ones, not macular ones) then targeted PRP may well be useful as there will be normal areas of retina that you will want to avoid. Widefield OCT-A, should that be available and of sufficient quality, might be an alternative, though this is not common at present outside one of the main teaching centres. If performing these tests would result in a delay, then it might well be best to make a value judgment about which areas of the retina need laser and to crack on with it.

If no neovascularisation occurs, follow up every 3 months until either the clinical signs of RVO disappear or 2 years have passed, whichever comes sooner, is a reasonable plan. Should neovascularisation occur and laser applied, then if the new vessels are then seen to shrink, the situation stabilises, and you are happy with the amount of laser applied in that it isn't homeopathic or has large gaps of gaping nothingness, then after monitoring every 3 months for 6 months it might well be possible to discharge the patient to the watchful eye of their community optometrist, should they be appropriately skilled and qualified in medical retina.

MACULAR OEDEMA

As with many other aspects of medical retina, there is guidance and then there is what is best for your patient. The person with ultimate moral responsibility is the clinician and not any faceless commissioner, manager or finance officer comfort-ably working from home somewhere. Guidelines do provide a good rule of thumb though, and while symptoms and visual acuity do not have a great bearing on whether to laser, the same is not true for macular oedema. If a patient is asymptom-atic or is very unbothered by their symptoms, then clearly the threshold for starting a course of treatment should be higher. If the vision is better than 0.18 LogMAR (or 6/9 Snellen), then it would be difficult to justify any treatment unless the patient is very bitterly complaining of symptoms of distortion or blur. If the vision is worse

than this but better than 1.20 LogMAR (6/96 Snellen), then symptoms don't necessarily need to be very significant at all to justify treatment, and an argument could
be made that even if no symptoms at all are present, then treatment is justified to
preserve the state of the macula long enough for recovery to occur. This argument is
weaker than with DMO, however, as in most cases, cystoid macular oedema (CMO)
related to RVO is self-limiting, whereas this is not the case with DMO under normal
circumstances.

At the other end of the scale, treatment could be justified, at least once to test
the water, if the vision is worse than 1.20 LogMAR but better than counting fingers (CF), if the patient is either very symptomatic, or if the affected eye is their
only good eye. If treatment is given at these extremes but the patient notices no
benefit, regardless of the effect on the OCT scan, then it is rarely worth repeating. Obviously, a proper go should be given; at least three anti-VEGF injections
at properly spaced intervals (slipped appointments due to an inadequate booking
system do not count) or a single dexamethasone injection (Ozurdex) should be
enough to know. Do not listen to industry-sponsored personalities who claim you
should always inject forever to truly know the truth. This is not in your patient's
best interests at all.

Within those visual boundaries, symptoms are less important and depending on
whether the patient is pseudophakic and without any history of glaucoma or ocular
hypertension, it is reasonable to start with Ozurdex, as this is good strong heavy
artillery that gets the job done. Because of the self-limiting nature of the condition,
Ozurdex suits CMO secondary to RVO better than DMO. If the patient is phakic
and younger than usual, and therefore not likely to need cataract surgery any time
soon, then anti-VEGF is best. This is also true if there is a history of glaucoma. The
same rules apply then as apply to DMO; if, after three injections of anti-VEGF in a
treat-and-extend regime, the fluid hasn't budged, have a low threshold to switch to
Ozurdex (unless glaucoma is an issue). Regarding the choice of anti-VEGF, it again
depends on the stability of your system. If, as with most of Wales and probably
much of England, follow-up intervals and capacity are issues, then a long-acting
anti-VEGF agent such as faricimab would be best. If you are lucky and are blessed
with more capacity in your injection service than you know what to do with, then a
cheaper, weaker agent can be justified on the grounds of health economics, though it
is not ideal in the grand scheme of things.

When is treatment stopped? There are two main criteria: when the fluid has
dried away and does not return, or it is proven not to be useful at all. As collateral development and adaptation to the blockage can mean resolution, after each
Ozurdex injection 2 monthly follow-up appointments to check for return of fluid,
with an option for patients to call for an earlier appointment should they notice
any deterioration beforehand, is a sensible way forward. If a treat-and-extend anti-
VEGF regime has been chosen, then waiting for the patient to fall off the end
of the algorithm is best, and if after a few monitoring visits the fluid does not
return, then it might be that if the retinopathy is also stable, the patient can be
discharged to the diabetic eye screening programme or a suitably qualified optometrist in the absence of a screening programme. Regular audit of results and being
open to tweaks here and there to improve results is sacrosanct to running a good

service. The below flowchart provides a schematic you can follow from diagnosis to management.

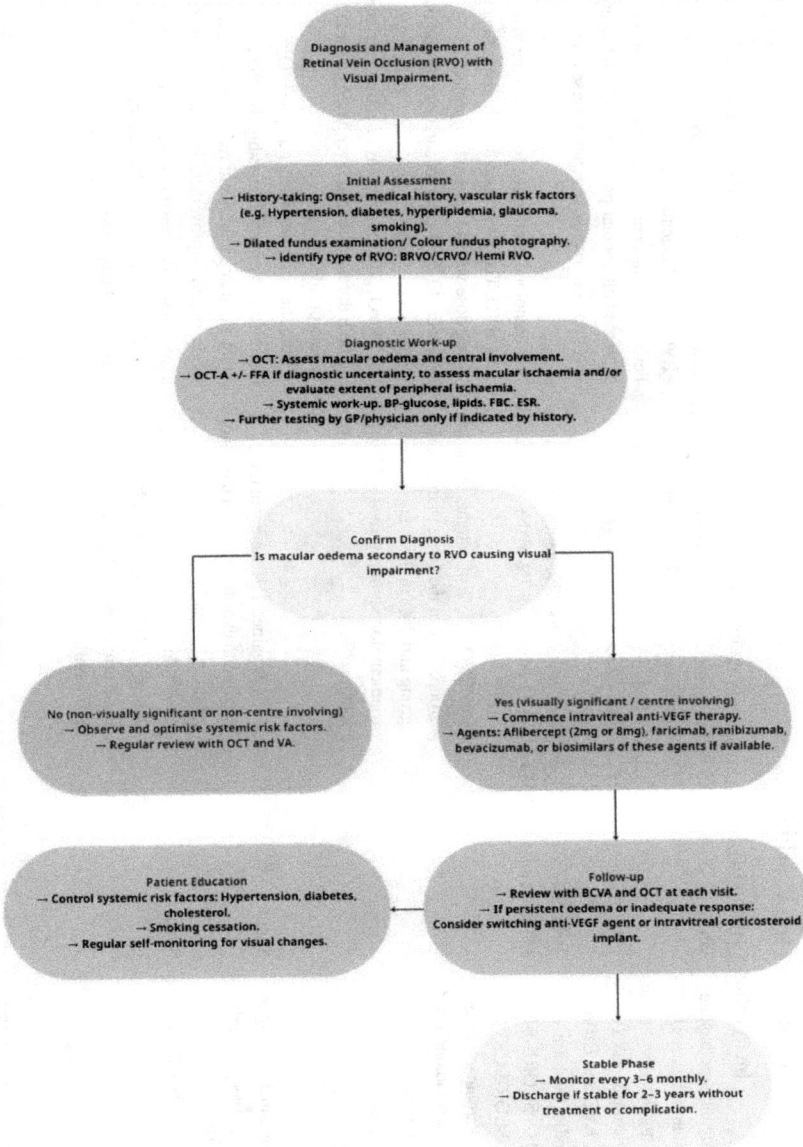

Diagnosis and Management of Retinal Vein Occlusion (RVO) with Visual Impairment.

Initial Assessment
→ History-taking: Onset, medical history, vascular risk factors (e.g. Hypertension, diabetes, hyperlipidemia, glaucoma, smoking).
→ Dilated fundus examination/ Colour fundus photography.
→ Identify type of RVO: BRVO/CRVO/ Hemi RVO.

Diagnostic Work-up
→ OCT: Assess macular oedema and central involvement.
→ OCT-A +/- FFA if diagnostic uncertainty, to assess macular ischaemia and/or evaluate extent of peripheral ischaemia.
→ Systemic work-up. BP-glucose, lipids. FBC. ESR.
→ Further testing by GP/physician only if indicated by history.

Confirm Diagnosis
Is macular oedema secondary to RVO causing visual impairment?

No (non-visually significant or non-centre involving)
→ Observe and optimise systemic risk factors.
→ Regular review with OCT and VA.

Yes (visually significant / centre involving)
→ Commence intravitreal anti-VEGF therapy.
→ Agents: Aflibercept (2mg or 8mg), faricimab, ranibizumab, bevacizumab, or biosimilars of these agents if available.

Patient Education
→ Control systemic risk factors: Hypertension, diabetes, cholesterol.
→ Smoking cessation.
→ Regular self-monitoring for visual changes.

Follow-up
→ Review with BCVA and OCT at each visit.
→ If persistent oedema or inadequate response: Consider switching anti-VEGF agent or intravitreal corticosteroid implant.

Stable Phase
→ Monitor every 3–6 monthly.
→ Discharge if stable for 2–3 years without treatment or complication.

Christiana Says...
Can we be more predictive in the management of macular oedema secondary to RVO? By this point, we know that mild macular oedema associated with RVO may resolve spontaneously, but many eyes require treatment to achieve optimal visual outcomes. Table 7.3 illustrates the effect of different treatments on macular oedema

TABLE 7.3
The Pivotal Trials for Therapies in the World of RVO

Study Name	Intervention	Comparator	Primary Outcome	Practice Implication
GENEVA	0.7 mg dexamethasone implant (Ozurdex) 0.35 mg dexamethasone implant (Ozurdex) For CRVO and BRVO	Sham	At 6 months, 41% achieved a ≥ 15 letter gain compared to 23% in the sham group Peak effect	Established Ozurdex as an effective therapy for RVO-related macular oedema Fewer injections compared to intravitreal anti-VEGF Increased intraocular pressure (IOP) and cataract progression were significant adverse events (6)
SCORE	2 parallel randomized trials – SCORE-BRVO • -SCORE-CRVO • - Participants received triamcinolone 1 mg or 4 mg	Grid laser for BRVO Observation for CRVO	For CRVO, 26–27% gained ≥ 15 letters at 12 months vs 7% in the observation arm For BRVO – 35% of patients in the laser group, 27% in the 1-mg triamcinolone group and 26% in the 4-mg triamcinolone group gained ≥ 15 letters	Triamcinolone is effective for improving visual acuity in CRVO. The 1-mg dose had similar efficacy to the 4-mg dose with a better safety profile. However, 40–60% cataract surgery rate and increased IOP. For BRVO, grid laser was as effective as triamcinolone in both doses, with grid laser having a more favorable safety profile. Set the stage for steroid therapy in RVO
BRAVO	Ranibizumab 0.3 mg or 0.5 mg every 4 weeks for BRVO	Sham	55–61% gained ≥ 15 letters in the ranibizumab arm vs 29% in the sham group at 6 months	Ranibizumab established as highly effective in BRVO with rapid and significant reduction in macular oedema and improvement in visual acuity (7)
CRUISE	As above for CRVO	Sham	47–48% in ranibizumab arm gained ≥ gained 15 letters or more. 17% of the sham arm gained ≥ 15 letters or more at 6 months	Ranibizumab demonstrated paid recovery of vision in CRVO-associated macular oedema and established as first-line therapy (8)

(Continued)

TABLE 7.3 (CONTINUED)
The Pivotal Trials for Therapies in the World of RVO

Study Name	Intervention Comparator		Primary Outcome	Practice Implication
COPERNICUS	2 mg Aflibercept every 4 weeks for CRVO	Sham	56% gained ≥15 letters vs 12% in sham at 6 months	Establishes Aflibercept as a choice of first-line therapy for CRVO (9)
Vibrant	Aflibercept 2 mg every 4 weeks for BRVO	Macular laser	52.7% gained 15 letters or more vs 26.7% in the laser arm; Mean ETDRS gain: +17 letters vs + 6.9 letters	Aflibercept established as superior to macular laser in BRVO-related macular oedema. (10)
BALATON and COMINO	Faricimab	Aflibercept every 4 weeks (11)	Mean gain in BCVA of +16.8 in faricimab arm vs +17.5 in Aflibercept arm for BRVO at month 6; Mean gain of +16.9 in faricimab arm vs +17.3 in Aflibercept arm for CRVO at month 6	Established Faricimab as non-inferior to Aflibercept for RVO
QUASAR	Aflibercept 8 mg every 8 weeks after 3 loading doses OR every 8 weeks after 5 loading doses	Aflibercept every 4 weeks	At 36 weeks: Eylea 2 mg arm gained +17.8 letters; Eylea 8 mg with 3 monthly loading gained +17 letters; Eylea 8 mg with 5 monthly dosing gained +19.8 letters	Demonstrates that Eylea 8 mg can achieve similar efficacy to 4 weekly Eylea 2 mg with fewer injections

in RVO. Some eyes may progress to atrophic changes at the macula with irreversible sight loss, a risk much lessened with adequate therapy. We are up-to-date with the progress in diagnosis using UWF-FP and UWF-FFA to better risk-stratify and prognosticate for our patients. We have also heard about the therapeutics we now have in our toolkit; intravitreal injections of anti-VEGF, steroids and occasionally adjunct macular laser in some cases. What evidence informs our current treatment paradigm? Can we predict which patients will respond best to different therapy classes, and are there any paradigm shifts on the horizon?

Early preclinical and clinical studies implicated VEGF as a major factor in the pathogenesis of RVO. Elevated levels of VEGF-A have been detected in ocular fluids in patients with CRVO and BRVO and correlate with the severity of macular oedema, possibly more strongly than we see in neovascular AMD and DMO. In addition, head-to-head trials comparing intravitreal anti-VEGF and intravitreal dexamethasone have demonstrated the superiority of anti-VEGF therapy (COMRADE-B, COMRADE-C and COMO trials (12–14), all of which are industry sponsored), while others failed to demonstrate the non-inferiority of intravitreal dexamethasone. The increased incidence of cataract progression, raised intraocular pressure (IOP), and in the United Kingdom, the accessibility of anti-VEGF treatment in the design of our services, means that anti-VEGF therapy is often the first-line treatment for macular oedema secondary to RVO. In terms of which anti-VEGF therapy to use, the LEAVO study, which compared bevacizumab, Aflibercept and ranibizumab for CRVO, demonstrated that Aflibercept is non-inferior to ranibizumab and may reduce injection burden, whilst bevacizumab did not meet the non-inferiority margin but was the most cost-effective (15).

A proportion of patients (30–50%) experience frequently recurrent or persistent macular oedema despite treatment with intravitreal anti-VEGF therapy. This may indicate the influence of alternative mechanisms beyond suppression of VEGF. In these cases, inflammatory proteins and cytokines such as interleukin 6 and 8, ICAM-I and others may play an important role, and treatment with corticosteroids such as intravitreal dexamethasone may help improve outcomes.

It would be desirable to identify eyes that would benefit from early switching to intravitreal corticosteroids where appropriate. A 'biomarker' is a characteristic that is objectively measured and evaluated as an indicator of normal biological activity, pathogenic processes or responses to therapeutic intervention. OCT biomarkers are particularly desirable as they are widely accessible, non-invasive and can be repeated frequently. Studies suggest hyperreflective foci, intraretinal cysts within the ganglion cell layer, disorganisation of the inner retinal layer, and disorganisation of the ellipsoid zone may be biomarkers that can identify eyes that may have an improved outcome with early intravitreal steroids, but larger studies are needed to validate these hypotheses are needed.

What about the future? RVO is rarely the main focus of therapeutic development. In most cases, therapeutic agents are developed and explored in neovascular AMD or DMO and then RVO is investigated as a secondary indication. Nevertheless, there remains unmet need in people diagnosed with RVO including a high burden of treatment with first-line anti-VEGF therapy. The recent approval of faricimab and Eylea 8 mg as second-generation anti-VEGF therapies with a focus on durability is a small step forward. Down the pike, we have novel mechanisms targeting VEGF C and D, tyrosine-kinase inhibitors and Wnt-signaling agonists. These may deliver more durable and efficacious treatments for macular oedema in the future.

NEOVASCULAR GLAUCOMA AND OTHER PRESSURE ISSUES

There are two reasons why pressure rises in RVO patients, which is why any virtual clinic setup needs to have some sort of mechanism for measuring IOP at each appointment. The main reason this occurs is usually because of us. Because we have given an Ozurdex injection. For this reason, it is vital to follow up all patients who have had an Ozurdex injection 6 weeks afterwards for an IOP check and, of course, to see if it's worked. The good news is that this can be treated by giving Latanoprost under most circumstances, remembering that the injection wears off after 3 to 6 months anyway. Should more than latanoprost be needed to weather the post-Ozurdex pressure storm, and say Cosopt is added as well, then Ozurdex should be avoided in the future. Bear in mind that Ozurdex does *not* shut off the VEGF drive in the same way that a true anti-VEGF injection does; neovascularisation can develop and worsen after Ozurdex.

The most dangerous reason pressure can rise is, of course, neovascular glaucoma. It is up to us to catch this before it becomes an issue and to treat it with laser, and whilst it is most definitely true that services that have slipped appointments are much more likely to suffer increased rates of neovascular glaucoma (and lawsuits as a result), this is a recognised major complication of RVO anyhow and a certain amount of pragmatism and planning are required to cope with this reality. Patients should be warned about this possibility right from the outset, with treatment for rubeosis being billed as 'preventing a blind eye from becoming a painful blind eye'. This is mainly to offset false expectations, whereby patients who cannot see might expect some sort of improvement in their vision after PRP laser, and when this inevitably does not happen, they deem your treatment a 'failure' even if it is successful in preventing further development of neovascularisation. The patient must always be told if the treatment is a success; otherwise, how might they know?

Sometimes the pressure battle is lost. Despite all our best efforts, the pressure goes up and up and pain sets in. The usual thing that Medical Retina specialists do is add Latanoprost first, then Cosopt on top if the pressure is still high (unless there is some sort of contraindication to beta blockers), then iopidine if the pressure is *still* high, and then acetazolamide (Diamox) tablets 250 mg SR bd. Finally, when the disc is fully cupped, all else is failed and the horse has well and truly bolted, then the glaucoma team are contacted for help. This is obviously not good practice, and if the battle with pressure is being lost, it is far better to contact the glaucoma team early, before disaster has well and truly set in. Our job is to make sure the VEGF drive has been eliminated with as much PRP as possible and anti-VEGF injections if needed. If the angle is zipped closed, but there is still visual potential, then the glaucoma team might be able to save sight with a glaucoma drainage procedure. If the battle is lost and pain is the issue, then cyclodiode laser might be the only option left to stop the pain. Either way, this is the purview of the glaucoma team, and our job is to try to control the situation as much as we can and refer as soon as we know the battle is being lost. Don't go down fighting; ask another warrior for help. Then you can both go down together.

Christiana Says...

Remember that in the CVOS study, approximately 20% of eyes treated with prophylactic PRP still developed neovascularisation of the iris and/or angle. Therefore, identifying those at high risk with UWF-FFA is still important. Treatment with anti-VEGF does not appear to modify the underlying risk of iris and/or angle neovascularisation, but rather shifts the timeline (16). As such, monitoring these eyes closely after cessation of anti-VEGF therapy remains important. The RCOphth guidance advises monitoring BRVO for 2 years after the last treatment before consideration for discharge, and 3 years for CRVO. It would be wise to assess the level of ischaemia before discharge and consider prophylactic PRP if significant. If there are trustworthy community partners present (such as WGOS4 practitioners with the higher certification in medical retina), then discharge much earlier than this is an option, though it could well be argued that is not true 'discharge' in the traditional sense.

AFTERWORD

RVO is very similar to diabetic eye disease, but it is not identical. It is friendlier by and large, and not a chronic condition in the same way as diabetes is. The key is to prepare the patient for potential complications and to temper expectations from an early stage. Better that your patient is pleasantly surprised rather than unexpectedly disappointed.

REFERENCES

1. Hayreh SS et al. BRVO: Natural history of visual outcome. JAMA Ophthalmol. 2014; 132(1)13:22.
2. Green WR et al. CRVO: Central retinal vein occlusion: a prospective histopathologic study of 29 eyes in 28 cases. Trans Am Ophthalmol Soc. 1981:79:371–422.
3. Dinah C, Chang A, Lee J, Li WW, Singh R, Wu L, Wong D, Saffar I. What is occluding our understanding of retinal vein occlusion? Ophthalmol Ther. 2024; 13(12):3025–3034. doi: 10.1007/s40123-024-01042-6.
4. Nicholson L, Vazquez-Alfageme C, Patrao NV, Triantafyllopolou I, Bainbridge JW, Hykin PG, Sivaprasad S. Retinal nonperfusion in the posterior pole is associated with increased risk of neovascularization in central retinal vein occlusion. Am J Ophthalmol. 2017; 182:118–125. doi: 10.1016/j.ajo.2017.07.015.
5. Baseline and early natural history report: The central vein occlusion study. Arch Ophthalmol. 1993; 111(8):1087–1095. doi: 10.1001/archopht.1993.01090080083022.
6. Haller JA et al. Dexamethasone intravitreal implant in patients with macular oedema related to branch or central retinal vein occlusion: Twelve-month study results. Ophthalmology. 2011; 118(12):2453–2460.
7. Campochiaro PA et al. Ranibizumab for macular oedema following branch retinal vein occlusion: 6 month primary end-point results of a phase 3 study. Ophthalmology. 2010; 117(6):1102–1112.
8. Campochiaro PA et al. Ranibizumab for macular oedema following central retinal vein occlusion: 6 month primary end-point results of a phase 3 study. Ophthalmology. 2010; 117(6):1124–1133.

9. Heier JS et al. Intravitreal aflibercept injection for macular oedema due to central retinal vein occlusion: The COPERNICUS study. Ophthalmology. 2012; 119(5):1024–1032.

10. Campochiaro PA et al. Randomized trial of vascular endothelial growth factor trap-eye for macular oedema secondary to branch retinal vein occlusion: The VIBRANT study. Ophthalmology. 2015; 122(3):538–544.

11. Danzig CJ et al. Efficacy, safety and durability of faricimab in macular oedema due to retinal vein occlusion: 72-week results from the BALATON and COMINO trials. Ophthalmology. 2024; 131(5):1024–1032.

12. Hattenbach LO, Feltgen N, Bertelmann T, Schmitz-Valckenberg S, Berk H, Eter N, Lang GE, Rehak M, Taylor SR, Wolf A, Weiss C, Paulus EM, Pielen A, Hoerauf H; COMRADE-B Study Group. Head-to-head comparison of ranibizumab PRN versus single-dose dexamethasone for branch retinal vein occlusion (COMRADE-B). Acta Ophthalmol. 2018; 96(1):e10–e18. doi: 10.1111/aos.13381.

13. Hoerauf H, Feltgen N, Weiss C, Paulus EM, Schmitz-Valckenberg S, Pielen A, Puri P, Berk H, Eter N, Wiedemann P, Lang GE, Rehak M, Wolf A, Bertelmann T, Hattenbach LO; COMRADE-C Study Group. Clinical efficacy and safety of ranibizumab versus dexamethasone for Central Retinal Vein Occlusion (COMRADE C): A European Label Study. Am J Ophthalmol. 2016; 169:258–267. doi: 10.1016/j.ajo.2016.04.020.

14. Bandello F, Augustin A, Tufail A, Leaback R. A 12-month, multicenter, parallel group comparison of dexamethasone intravitreal implant versus ranibizumab in branch retinal vein occlusion. Eur J Ophthalmol. 2018; 28(6):697–705. doi: 10.1177/1120672117750058. Epub 2018 Apr 9.

15. Hykin P, Prevost AT, Sivaprasad S, Vasconcelos JC, Murphy C, Kelly J, Ramu J, Alshreef A, Flight L, Pennington R, Hounsome B, Lever E, Metry A, Poku E, Yang Y, Harding SP, Lotery A, Chakravarthy U, Brazier J. Intravitreal ranibizumab versus aflibercept versus bevacizumab for macular oedema due to central retinal vein occlusion: The LEAVO non-inferiority three-arm RCT. Health Technol Assess. 2021; 25(38):1–196. doi: 10.3310/hta25380.

16. Brown DM, Wykoff CC, Wong TP, Mariani AF, Croft DE, Schuetzle KL; RAVE Study Group. Ranibizumab in preproliferative (ischemic) central retinal vein occlusion: The rubeosis anti-VEGF (RAVE) trial. Retina. 2014; 34(9):1728–1735. doi: 10.1097/IAE.0000000000000191.

8 Central Serous Chorioretinopathy

There are some conditions that cause both the patient and ophthalmologist pain; this is one of them – perhaps the main one. A referral will come from a primary care optometrist mentioning central serous chorioretinopathy (CSCR), and your heart will sink. Sometimes a new optometrist will unwittingly cause a bigger problem for you than intended by referring the patient as a 'priority' patient or even an urgent case. CSCR is categorically not urgent nor a priority case. It is a heartsink of doom. When these referrals come in by letter, there is only one determination to be made here: Can the diagnosis be trusted?

IS IT REALLY CSCR?

Looking at the referral is the most important step. If the optometrist is referring a patient as a case of CSCR, then it is best to look at the age of the patient, the details present in the letter, and the visual acuity. A nice clear referral where the patient is young, or at least younger than 60 years of age, has typical symptoms of visual blurring centrally and the vision is 0.18 LogMAR (6/9) or better is great. If the optometrist mentions CSCR directly and hints that an optical coherence tomography (OCT) scan has been done, this is a huge bonus, and if the letter mentions that there is specifically subretinal fluid (SRF), then this is a gold standard referral indeed. If all these factors are present, then you can happily and confidently grade the referral as 'routine' on the grading form, which has the maximum 26-week referral-to-clinic target. There is no usefulness in bringing the patient in any sooner; in fact, the longer the better because it gives you hope that it might have cleared up spontaneously in the time that it takes them to come to clinic. The incidence of new disease is 1 per 10,000 people per year, with one-third recurring at some time, and resolution typically taking between 3 and 6 months. Men are approximately six times more commonly affected than women, and visual acuity tends not to be very adversely affected, with an average presenting acuity of 0.18 LogMAR.

If there is any doubt, the referring diagnosis must be questioned. If the patient is older than 60 years of age, if the symptoms are atypical, or if blood or intraretinal fluid (IRF) is mentioned, then raise an eyebrow. If the visual acuity is seriously affected, then raise both eyebrows. Could this be neovascular age-related macular degeneration (nAMD), retinal vein occlusion (RVO), or diabetic eye disease? Could it be something else again? If there is doubt, then you cannot grade the referral as routine. With a heavy heart, you must bring them to clinic sooner for assessment. If a community referral refinement scheme for nAMD exists, then you could potentially send it via that scheme so that a properly skilled optometrist, qualified specifically in medical retina, can take a look. If anything other than CSCR is indeed

DOI: 10.1201/9781003628309-8

present, then they can be trusted to send the patient via the proper route, and if the heartsink CSCR is indeed present, then you can more confidently grade the patient as routine. If the letter specifically mentions stress and urges you to see the patient as soon as possible, then if anything, this is an indication not to do so. You won't be rewarded.

WHAT IS CSCR?

CSCR is a curious condition that even now is not properly understood. There are many theories, but these do not really alter what you do and are not really that interesting, and so won't be mentioned in detail here. In fact, the only thing that needs to be known roughly is that the adrenal gland atop the kidney produces adrenaline when stressed and also produces steroids needed for the body to function. A side effect of too much adrenal activity, be it through steroids or adrenaline, is that vascular permeability is affected and fluid can accumulate in the space between the retina and the retinal pigment epithelium (RPE).

The retina is like the polders of the Netherlands, essentially below sea level, with the RPE cells being like eternally turning windmills charged with keeping the retina dry by constantly pumping out fluid. Any breach in the dyke or defect in the pumping action, and the fluid simply flows back in again. Therefore, the fluid is subretinal first and foremost. Could this be true? Possibly. It's good to have some sort of narrative to tell patients, and this is as good as any. Patients don't like to hear 'nobody knows', and there is something noble in being told they have too much adrenaline as they are just working so hard. You read it here, so you could technically say that you saw it in a book.

There are two main causes – steroids and stress. The adrenal gland producing excessive steroids of its own is rare indeed. Far more commonly, a patient with CSCR will be taking steroids of their own – exogenous steroids via tablets for some other medical condition, on the skin in the form of a cream, via injections into joints, or even in sprays up the nose or into the lungs. If the patient denies taking any steroid (and is a youngish male especially) in any form, then it is worth looking them directly in the eye and stating that not all steroids are legal and sometimes illegal steroids can be sourced in gyms, for example, and then seeing what happens. If the patient looks straight back and states simply that they have not taken any steroids, legal or illegal, then they are probably telling the truth, but if they look at the floor or ceiling or mumble something incoherent, then you have your answer.

Stress is the other main thing of note, pummeling away at the adrenal gland, squeezing it dry of all sorts of substances. Unlike steroids, patients readily admit stress. At the end of the day, everyone is stressed. Being stressed means you work hard. You care. But this knowledge is also utterly useless because you can do nothing about it. If it were easy to stop stress, everyone would do so spontaneously. There are type A and type B personalities: stressed and highly strung and relaxed and laidback, with CSCR being said to be far commoner in the former. Again, this is not useful from a practical purpose because one cannot simply change their personality on a whim. So the only truly alterable factor is the steroid aspect.

Christiana Says...

Researchers also hypothesise that CSCR may be due to choroidal venous overload in common with diseases such as vortex vein occlusion, carotid-cavernous sinus fistula, peripapillary pachychoroid syndrome, and spaceflight-associated neuro-ocular syndrome. This unified hypothesis provides a framework to deepen our understanding of the processes involved in the pathophysiology of CSCR. A deeper understanding is certainly needed, as you will come to see, given the limited treatment options available and resulting visual impairment in chronic cases.

DIAGNOSIS

First, the patient has to fall into the correct demographic; youngish (less than 60 years of age), with a history of some central scotoma or distortion but generally good visual acuity (0.18 LogMAR (6/9) or better). The absolute key, of course, is the OCT scan, as with so much else in the world of medical retina. There will be a nicely symmetrical dome of SRF with some sort of pigment epithelial detachment (PED) somewhere under the dome (see Figure 8.1). This PED can be very small or larger, but it will be serous and 'tidy', as in simple but not complex. If the PED is solid, no PED present at all, or the PED has multiple peaks and troughs, then a choroidal neovascular membrane (CNVM) might be present. In fact, nAMD is the main differential diagnosis, and an OCT angiography (OCT-A) is always a useful non-invasive test. This is especially the case if the patient is not young or there is some sort of unusual feature present.

Confusion comes if the CSCR is persistent. If the patient is unlucky and the fluid remains over a long period, the OCT appearance can get increasingly distorted. Normally, there is no IRF, but with enough time, IRF starts to appear and then perhaps even becomes dominant. The outer retinal border is normally crisp and straight, but again, with enough time, the border can become ragged. The key here is then confirming CSCR with fundus autofluorescence (FAF).

FAF is a test that is an 'RPE-ogram' of sorts and looks at the health of the RPE by measuring the natural fluorescent pigments that exist within the cells. CSCR is

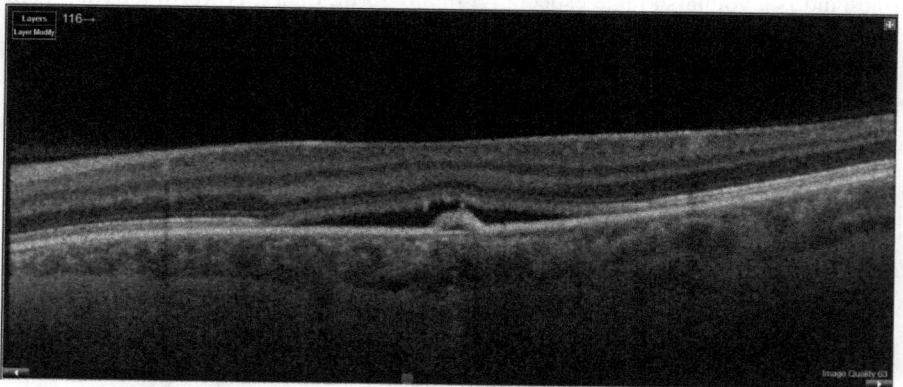

FIGURE 8.1 Central serous chorioretinopathy (CSCR) with pigment epithelial detachment (PED).

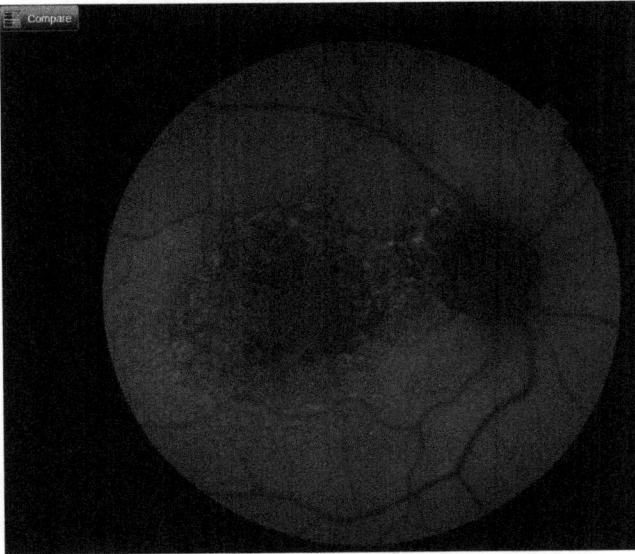

FIGURE 8.2 A fundus autofluorescence (FAF) image of a patient with CSCR.

distinctive in that the RPE is degraded across a wide area under the macula with gravity-derived tracking lines leading inferiorly from the leaky area. On FAF, this RPE dysfunction, including tracking lines, can be clearly seen, whereas it is very difficult to see with the naked eye alone (see Figure 8.2). Even when the OCT might show complete resolution of the fluid, the FAF tells no lie. It will never be normal again. If the OCT and history are obvious, then of course an autofluorescence image is not needed, but it really comes into its own if the diagnosis is in doubt.

Traditionally, a fundus fluorescein angiogram (FFA) can show distinctive images with patterns that frequently come up in exams but are increasingly irrelevant in real clinical life. These include the smokestack image, where the dye leaks out in a way reminiscent of the chimneys of the industrial revolution, billowing smoke that swirls in the wind. The so-called ink blot is the other classic pattern, where a small blob of leaking becomes a bigger blob and then becomes a bigger blob again. It is relatively rare to perform routine FFA now with CSCR suspects, but should you do so, these are the things of which to be aware; however, OCT and FAF are far more important and relevant. Table 8.1 displays the features of CSCR on various images.

There are also atypical variants of CSCR that can cause diagnostic dilemmas. Bullous CSCR cases are associated with very large, dome-shaped serous retinal detachment and can mimic rhegmatogenous retinal detachments. RPE tears are prevalent in this variant of CSCR. Some cases can present as bilateral bullous serous detachments and/or subretinal fibrin mimicking diseases such as Vogt–Koyanagi–Harada (VKH) syndrome. Careful history taking, including systemic evaluation and multimodal imaging, is useful here to prevent inappropriate use of steroids, which may exacerbate the whole problem.

TABLE 8.1

Features of Central Serous Chorioretinopathy on Multimodal Imaging

OCT	Enhanced-depth Imaging OCT (EDI-OCT)	Fundus Autofluorescence	FFA	Indocyanine Green Angiography (ICGA)	OCT-A
Serous retinal detachment	Thickened choroid	Hypoautofluorescence in areas of SRF (acute)	Gradual, well-defined expansion of hyperfluorescent spot (inkblot, classic) Smoke stack pattern: vertical expanding column of dye	Mid-phase: multifocal choroidal hyperpermeability	Attenuation or absence of choriocapillaris flow signal beneath areas of subretinal detachment
Pigment epithelial detachment	Dilated choroidal vessels in Haller's layer	Surrounding hyperautofluorescence	Window defects in areas of RPE atrophy (typically chronic)	Dilated choroidal vessels	Flow signal beneath RPE indicating CNVM
Elongated photoreceptor outer segments (especially chronic cases)		Diffuse areas of hyper- and hypoautofluoresence (chronic and can be gravitational)	Multiple foci of leakage	Delayed choroidal filling	
				Late staining of choroidal vessels	

Lastly, in the ultimate twisty twist, as a complication of chronic CSCR, a secondary neovascular membrane can develop. This is particularly ironic because the main differential diagnosis is indeed a CNVM and the OCT images can become increasingly similar as chronicity takes hold. If OCT-A reveals an obvious membrane and there is any hint of blood present, then the diagnosis is certain, with FAF revealing characteristically degraded RPE. You might argue that it matters not if the CNVM is due to, say, nAMD and simply resembles CSCR, or whether it is a secondary membrane due to chronic chorioretinopathy, but it does very much so. This is mainly because CNVM can be treated in the normal way mentioned in Chapter 4, but if the CNVM is due to CSCR, then all the injections in all the world won't clear up all the fluid. This is because anti-vascular endothelial growth factor (anti-VEGF) injections do nothing for CSCR, nothing at all, and the fact that a membrane develops does not mean that suddenly the chorioretinopathy disappears. If two taps are left on in your bath and the bath starts flooding, closing one tap will in some way reduce the water pressure, but with the other still flowing, water will still pour. All the pressure in all of the world on closing the tap that is already closed won't affect the tap still open. Therefore, the normal nAMD algorithms break down, as aiming for complete dryness is impossible in these chronic cases, or at least improbable.

MANAGEMENT

Masterly inactivity is key. Less is more. See new referrals routinely, and there is a good chance things will have settled by the time they reach you. There are few things worse than seeing a patient with CSCR in clinic right after referral and then saying, 'okay, you have this; let's see you in 3 months to see if it's gone'. If by the time you see the patient it is already gone, then you can discharge them right away with advice. Patients don't like being told there is no easy treatment. CSCR patients are anxious, and Google is the refuge of such folk. The fact that there are so many treatments available is a testament to the fact that none of them do anything. Eplerenone, melatonin, rifampicin and many more have been touted as treatments. They are not. The only good they do, if any, is to calm the patient down by convincing them that 'something is being done', with perhaps the reduction in stress causing some sort of resolution. This is not good medicine though and should not be done.

The only true treatment that does anything is photodynamic therapy (PDT). This is when verteporfin is injected into the vein and a diode laser is shone on the macula, which nicely cooks the leaking spot. Compared to any other treatment, this is the only thing that does anything much, although there has been a problem of late with obtaining verteporfin due to various manufacturing issues and price fluctuations. There was a period when verteporfin was being reserved exclusively for use in ocular oncology. As a result, many centres that used to perform PDT therapy stopped, and since some increased availability of verteporfin has now occurred, some services have simply not picked up the baton again. There are, therefore, places throughout the country where, to all intents and purposes, access to PDT does not exist as it did before this manufacturing issue came up. In managing the difficult condition that is CSCR, not only is one hand tied behind our back, but we now have both hands and both feet tied with no immediate rescue in sight. If you have access to PDT count yourself lucky.

But when do you perform PDT, or indeed refer for PDT if it is undertaken elsewhere? After a lot of doing nothing. Doing nothing and telling the patient to avoid steroids and stress. If the patient at their first clinic appointment, despite having graded the referral routine and the passage of several months, still has fluid present, the next question to ask is whether the symptoms are improving or worsening. If they are improving, then you can breathe a sigh of relief and ask the patient about steroids and stress (highlighting avoidance of both) before handing them a leaflet and giving them an appointment in another 3 months, or longer again if possible, to 'check that it has improved'. If it has, they can then be discharged. The SRF does indeed disappear, but the associated PED usually remains, and waiting for that to go would be purposeless. Once the SRF is gone, you can discharge them back to their optometrist.

Should the patient worsen between the first appointment and the second, then the patient will be expecting something to be done. You have the option to ask more sternly about any hidden steroid use or undisclosed stress, and if this buys you another 3 months, great, but if not, then an option is to perform an FFA to see if there are any laserable lesions. If a single hot spot highlights itself far enough away from the fovea, usually half a disc diameter away at the very least, then you can consider tickling it with a very light laser to see what happens. This would be the same laser as that used for panretinal photocoagulation (PRP), though at a diameter of only 100 microns and power of 100 mW. Do not leave a mark, and do not shoot multiple times. Keep the FFA image on screen so you can map exactly where to shoot. Measure twice, but cut once. Does this work? Possibly. It cannot be dismissed. Usually, there is no specific lesion to shoot, or if there is, it is too close to the fovea, but sometimes there is a target that is shootable. After undertaking this laser, you can then follow up with the patient in 3 months to 'see if it's worked'.

If it is unshootable or does not work but remains stubbornly resistant, then it might be time for PDT, and should you be in a region where this is simply unobtainable, then an awkward conversation with the patient needs to be had, followed by angry emails to hospital management pleading for this situation to be fixed. Perhaps by filling out a patient funding request, the patient could be transferred to a region that does; you will receive a letter a few months later from the receiving hospital thanking you for the referral but informing you that PDT was not done in the end as it had resolved of its own accord. At this point, the patient will be re-referred to you from their optometrist with a recurrence. Such is the nature of CSCR. If, however, you are lucky enough to work in a unit that can undertake this directly, then you can actually do something to help the patient. Under no circumstances should treatments that are known not to work be given just for the sake of 'doing something', even if a patient turns up with a sheaf of Google printouts pressuring you for a whole host of things.

TABLE 8.2
Important Studies in CSCR Treatment

	VICI (1)	PLACE (2)
Authors	Lotery et al.	
Design	Randomised quadruple-blind placebo-controlled 25 mg eplerenone daily for 1 week, then 50 mg daily for 12 months versus placebo	Half-dose PDT vs high-density subthreshold micropulse laser
Results	No difference in BCVA at 12 months No anatomical benefit	67.2% of PDT-treated eyes demonstrated no SRF vs 28.8% of micropulse-treated eyes
Interpretation	Not superior to placebo	Half-dose PDT superior to micropulse laser

Christiana Says...
The natural history of CSCR, which includes spontaneous resolution and a relapsing and remitting course, poses specific challenges when designing a clinical trial to determine the clinical efficacy of therapies for this condition. Indeed, the literature is littered with case reports and case series of a wide variety of interventions for CSCR demonstrating benefit. Very few of them have stood the test of a robustly designed randomised controlled trial (RCT) (see Table 8.2). Because most cases of acute CSCR may recover spontaneously within 4 months, observation is the first-line approach. Considering the relatively good visual prognosis, any treatment for chronic CSCR must be evidence-based and safe. Overall, PDT at reduced settings (half-dose or half-fluence) remains the most robustly supported proven intervention for chronic CSCR, with anatomical resolution of fluid in two-thirds of patients compared to one-quarter with micropulse laser and more patients again achieving five letters or more of best corrected visual acuity (BCVA) gain.

PROGNOSIS

If a patient has a single episode of CSCR that quickly resolves, then the prognosis is excellent. This is doubly so if the episode was linked to a period of intense stress or high-dose oral steroid usage that is unlikely to be repeated. If the CSCR is recurrent, however, with time and chronicity, the outlook declines as the RPE starts to deteriorate and the retina itself becomes increasingly waterlogged and cystic. If secondary CNVM occurs, then the prognosis dips further, with injections of an anti-VEGF agent being a rearguard action to delay the enemy until it finally overwhelms us. It buys time but does not effect a cure. It is important to be open and honest with your patient about this from the outset because otherwise, they will think your treatments have failed when in fact they were never designed to win outright, only slow things down. Informing the patient's general practitioner if steroid is the cause to avoid steroids as much as possible can be useful, but otherwise, seeing patients with CSCR is unsatisfying and in the current climate of lack of access to PDT quite depressing, for both patient and doctor. This is where your skill as a modern communication expert, taught so thoroughly in medical schools at present, will really come into its own.

REFERENCES

1. Lotery A, Sivaprasad S, O'Connell A, Harris RA, Culliford L, Ellis L, Cree A, Madhusudhan S, Griffiths H, Ellis L, Chakravarthy U, Peto T, Rogers CA, Reeves BC; VICI Study Group. Eplerenone for chronic central serous chorioretinopathy in patients with active, previously untreated disease for more than 4 months (VICI): A randomised, double-blind, placebo-controlled trial. Lancet. 2020; 395(10220):294–303.
2. van Rijssen TJ, van Dijk EHC, Fauser S, Breukink MB, Dijkman G, Peters PJH, Keunen JEE, Blanco-Garavito R, Souied EH, MacLaren RE, Downes SM, Hoyng CB, Boon CJF. Half-dose photodynamic therapy versus high-density subthreshold micropulse laser treatment in patients with chronic central serous chorioretinopathy: The PLACE trial. Ophthalmology. 2018; 125(10):1547–1555.

9 Inherited Retinal Dystrophies and Genetic Conditions

This book is for the coalface Medical Retina specialist, not the expert in a large teaching hospital working in an ivory tower. No set of conditions is treated so differently in ophthalmology at the humble district general hospital compared with a Centre of Excellence than this group of eye diseases. For this reason, many regular Medical Retina specialists are unfamiliar with the vast array of diseases that exist and don't know the best thing to do when faced with a new patient presenting with what might well be a genetic condition. We will provide step-by-step guidance for approaching these seemingly complex families of conditions. The first, of course, is to suspect that the condition affecting the patient in front of you is indeed genetic in nature.

WHEN TO SUSPECT AN EYE CONDITION IS GENETIC

This might seem like an easy thing, but it isn't difficult to be misled. Typically, if a youngish patient, as in younger than 60 years of age, presents with a bilateral eye condition that looks atypical for an obvious acquired disease, then this should be considered. There are different flavours of genetic medical retina conditions, but these can be separated into ones that predominantly affect the retina and others that predominantly affect the macula. Should the condition be serious, there is a high chance that clever paediatric ophthalmologists will have already diagnosed it and done all relevant genetic testing before they hit the age at which regular Medical Retina specialists become involved. This would include things such as X-linked retinoschisis, Best vitelliform macular dystrophy and some variants of Stargardt disease. There is nothing to do then, from a diagnostic perspective, and simply following patients and offering support when needed via certification of visual impairment, for example, is best.

History is key as well. If a patient mentions something akin to night blindness, nyctalopia, then this is important information. It is all too easy, however, to be so keen to diagnose an inherited condition that we ask in such a way that the patient's answer is biased. 'Can you see in the dark?' for example, will always result in 'no, of course not', as nobody can. Asking 'do you have more difficulties than most in dim light?' is infinitely more useful; an example may be in the cinema or at dusk.

If, however, patients present with symptoms in adulthood, it will fall on us to suspect the condition has a genetic component and to investigate accordingly. The younger the patient sitting in front of us, the easier suspicion will arise in us, but it is important to also have an open mind with older patients. Regarding predominantly macular dystrophies, if a younger patient than average has signs of what appears

DOI: 10.1201/9781003628309-9

to be macular degeneration, it is worth asking whether genetics might be responsible. This is doubly so if it is what appears to be geographic atrophy (GA) that is taking place. If there are flecks and patterns around the macula that look unusual, then do not be tempted to automatically assume the condition is degenerative. Other genetic conditions might present with a bull's eye maculopathy and be confused with hydroxychloroquine toxicity. Retinal conditions generally might involve pigmented peripheral lesions, classically described as 'bone spicule pigmentation', as they do give the impression of cut bone graininess-wise. Similarly, there might be more peripheral flecks and dots that don't look typical of anything degenerative and make the clinician immediately think of a genetic cause.

If the thought occurs to you, it is always useful to ask the patient if anyone else in the family has an eye condition and, if so, what it is. Disappointingly, more than a few patients do tend to answer that some random relative did indeed 'go totally blind', but that they are utterly unaware of what the diagnosis is, which means that, essentially, the information is not very useful because it could well be cataracts, glaucoma or something such as that. Lastly, whilst it can be argued by the pedantic that almost all eye conditions do, in fact, have a genetic element – macular degeneration, glaucoma and the like – what we refer to here are 'proper' genetic diseases that are inherited in a specific way (Mendelian inheritance), for which patients want to know the prognosis for them and their children.

SUBSETS OF CONDITIONS

There is no use in being able to name 300 different sorts of macular dystrophies unless you work in Moorfields, and even then, the value of knowing this sort of information is questionable. The lumper versus splitter debate here can be summarised as 'regular coalface clinicians need to lump, while the big units have the luxury of splitting'. There are myriad ways to look at different categories of conditions, and this is one:

1. Retinitis pigmentosa (sometimes called rod–cone dystrophy), including Usher syndrome
2. Stargardt variants affecting the peripheral retina (also called ABCA4 retinopathy by experts)
3. Choroideremia
4. Something else that doesn't neatly fit into these categories
   These are the four sorts of diagnoses into which predominantly retinal dystrophies can fall, with predominantly macular conditions falling into the following groups:

5. Cone–rod dystrophy
6. Best disease
7. Pattern dystrophy
8. Stargardt variants affecting the macula more
9. Things that get confused with macular degeneration, such as Sorsby and Doyne

Then there are conditions such as pseudoxanthoma elasticum (PXE); this will be discussed in the next chapter because it is a systemic condition and is sufficiently different from the above that it needs to be treated separately. Regarding traditional inherited macular and retinal conditions, the above groups are all you really need to know. There is no usefulness in day-to-day life of knowing all the pattern dystrophies for example, the things that can mimic macular degeneration (except to know that they exist) or the myriad conditions that cause peripheral dystrophies that aren't the big ones. If you're specifically interested, then great, but it doesn't really change management. Knowing the specific mutations involved might seem impressive, but has even less utility in life. The various categories can be distinguished by examination in the first instance.

EXAMINATION

This has been compared to a form of medical ornithology of sorts, as there are key features that can be picked out to shoehorn findings into one category over another. Let us take each one in turn.

Retinitis pigmentosa (RP) is an umbrella term for a group of conditions that end with the death of photoreceptors. Everything in life is a spectrum if you look hard enough, and RP can be described as a condition affecting rods more than cones or cones more than rods, which is the origin of the terms rod–cone and cone–rod dystrophies. In the more peripheral rod–cone dystrophy variant, the classic triad consists of peripheral bone spicule pigmentation, attenuated vessels and a waxy disc. The main thing that stands out is the first, and the pigmentation comes slowly over time, but has a distinctive fleck appearance with spikes and clumps (see Figure 9.1).

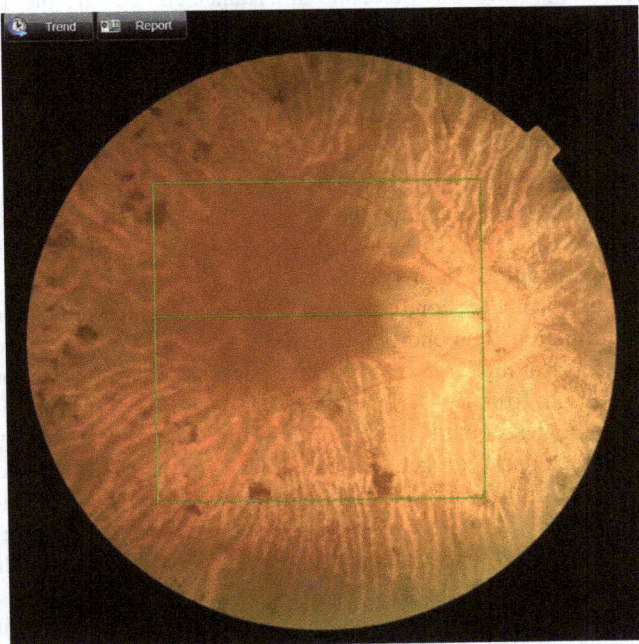

FIGURE 9.1 Retinitis pigmentosa (RP).

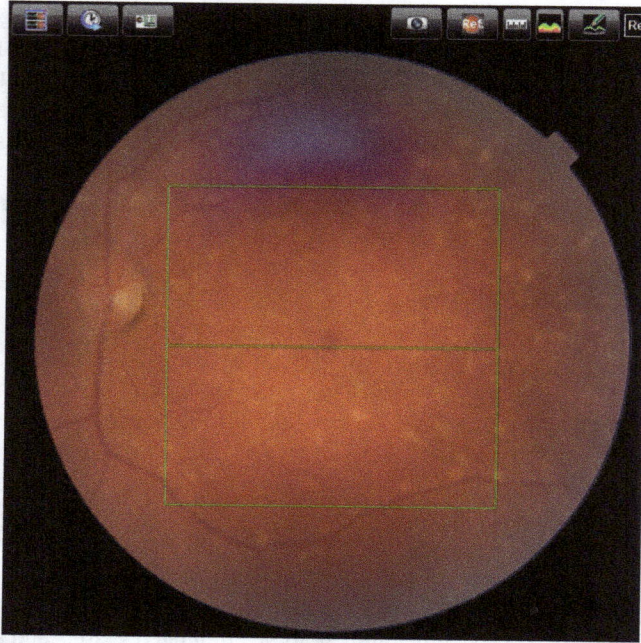

FIGURE 9.2   Stargardt disease affecting the retina predominantly.

Nyctalopia features prominently here, and inheritance can be variable. If the patient has RP and deafness, then it is specifically termed Usher syndrome, so it is worth asking about hearing.

Stargardt disease is more properly called ABCA4 retinopathy, named after the mutation itself, though Stargardt disease is still much more widely used and so will be used here too. The flecks here are less peripheral and yellowish in nature rather than pigmented and are described as 'pisciform', as in fish-like, but they rarely look anything like fish in reality. Sometimes the term 'fundus flavimaculatus', is used, though it is rarely useful to have many different names for the same condition. Figure 9.2 displays the fundus appearance in this condition. Inheritance is recessive.

Choroideremia is another condition that is distinctive enough to be readily recognised on examination. The choroid essentially starts to die away, and disappear completely, in fact, leaving large blank white spaces where the posterior sclera can be directly visualised, from the peripheries from a young age onwards. This eventually expands and coalesces until there is only a tiny island of normality located at the fovea, which then itself can get snuffed out later in life. Figure 9.3 demonstrates how this looks on examination. It is an X-linked recessive condition, which makes it a disease affecting almost entirely males. It is included because it is rare, but has its own category because it is so distinctive that it can be one of those spot diagnoses so beloved by certain clinical teachers.

Last in this category of inherited conditions chiefly affecting the retina over the macula, we have a basket of *everything else*. This basket includes such things as

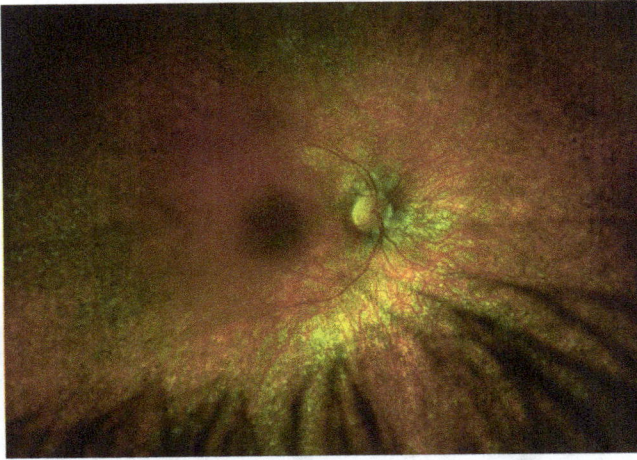

FIGURE 9.3   Choroideremia.

congenital stationary night blindness (CSNB), which is itself a basket of conditions that includes entities such as fundus albipunctatus, where there are white dots over the fundus; Oguchi disease, with its peculiar Mizuo-Nakamura phenomenon which, while interesting, is clinically irrelevant as you will never see a case of this in all your born days; and other conditions, again, with a seemingly normal-looking fundus. As the name suggests, these are stationary conditions; they do not progress and in that way are fundamentally different from true retinal dystrophies. However, they can look the same; a case in point is retinitis punctata albescens, which is indeed a progressive dystrophy, but because it features white dots all over the fundus looks similar to fundus albipunctatus. There is no great usefulness in regular clinicians knowing these things, as well as the myriad other conditions that it would take too long to list here. However, we should know that this basket of conditions exists, and whilst we ourselves don't understand them, we know how to investigate and pass them to someone who does.

Cone–rod dystrophy is the inverse, in a way, of RP, also called rod–cone dystrophy, where cones are more affected than rods. Cones see colour and are more central; there-fore, nyctalopia is less of a thing, but the macula and central vision are affected more. It isn't one condition, of course, and involves very many mutations and a spectrum of phenotypes that stretch from what looks like RP but with 'something mild going on at the macula', to normal peripheral retina with bull's eye maculopathy, to what appears to be indistinguishable from GA. Symptom-wise, there is a phenomenon called day-blindness, or more correctly hemeralopia, where people see much better in the dark than in the light. In practice, this is much more difficult to ask about than night blind-ness, but is said to be a feature of cone–rod dystrophy. Inheritance is variable.

Best disease is more properly called Best vitelliform macular dystrophy and has a juvenile form and an adult form. The juvenile form is the much more proper, much more official form, and is relatively easy to distinguish, as there are bilateral yellow-ish blobs at the maculae that over time break down into scarring, with progressive loss of vision. The term vitelliform comes from the Latin for egg yolk. With albumin being the egg white, though this is merely interesting and not of relevance here. Figure 9.4 demonstrates how a patient with Best disease looks on examination. The juvenile type is inherited in an autosomal dominant way, though the adult version is not. In fact, the adult version shouldn't really be put in this chapter at all, strictly speaking. It is a form of dry macular degeneration that phenotypically resembles true Best both on examination and on optical coherence tomography (OCT) scanning, but lacks the genetic and electrophysiology element and confusingly is oftentimes grouped under the next heading we will discuss, pattern dystrophy.

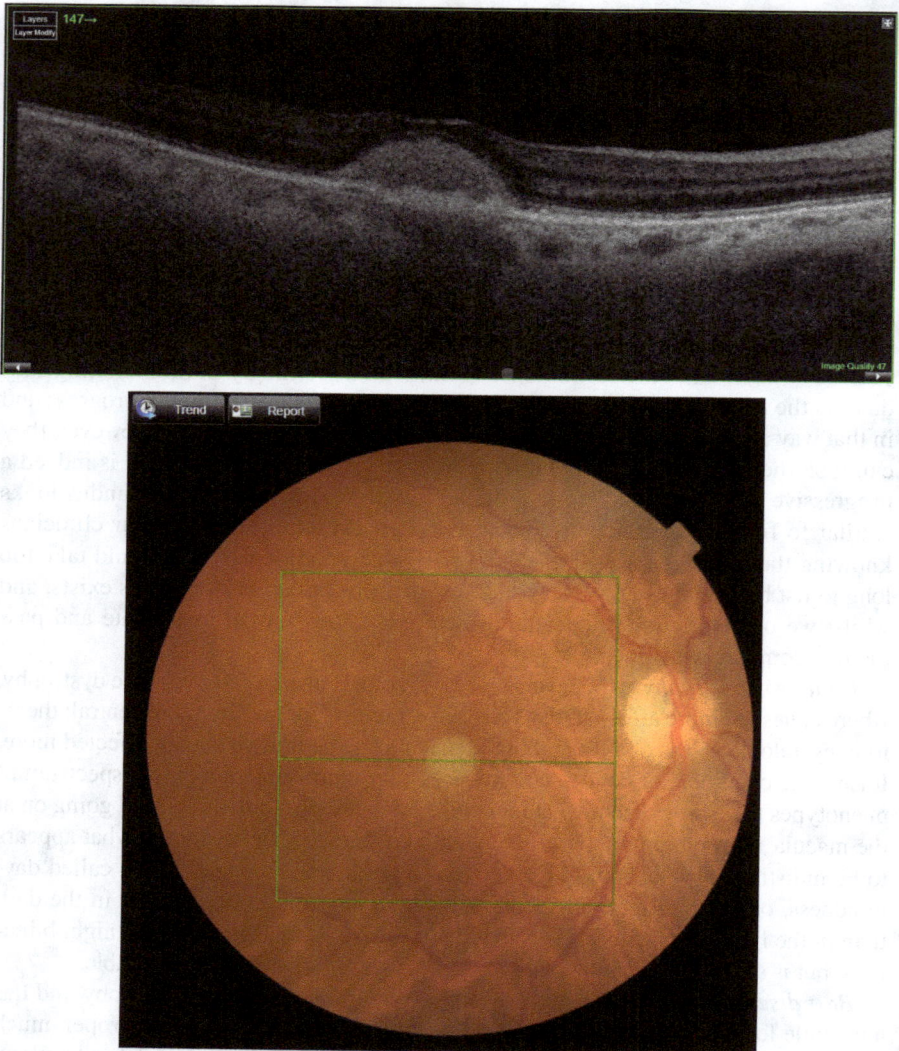

FIGURE 9.4   Best vitelliform macular dystrophy.

Pattern dystrophy is another umbrella term for a group of significantly varied conditions that affect the macula and includes, confusingly, adult-onset Best disease (otherwise known as adult-onset vitelliform dystrophy). In our opinion, this should not be grouped here, but we don't make the rules. The retinal pigment epithelium (RPE) is the layer most affected; other conditions that fall under this banner include butterfly-shaped pigment dystrophy, which does not resemble a butterfly in any way and rather a weirdly dendritic macular pigmentation, fundus pulverulentus, and other peculiarly named entities. Figure 9.5 displays a typical case of butterfly-shaped pigment dystrophy. There really is no need to memorise these names or how they look except to suspect that any peculiar pigmented patterns at the macula not typical of macular degeneration could, in fact, fall into the basket that is pattern dystrophy. The genetics are variable and confusing, but the important thing to note with all pattern dystrophies is that there can be systemic associations with conditions such as myotonic dystrophy, PXE and maternally inherited diabetes and deafness (MIDD). MIDD is a result of mitochondrial mutation and as such is why it is maternally inherited and also causes, well, diabetes and deafness. You won't diagnose these conditions based on the eye, by the way; they will almost always be diagnosed already. The point of mentioning them here is that patients mentioning these things in their history are more likely to have pattern dystrophy.

Stargardt disease, or ABCA4 retinopathy, is itself a form of umbrella term in a whole world of umbrellas. It was discussed above but is discussed here because there are variants, depending on where the mutation is on the ABCA4 gene, that affect the

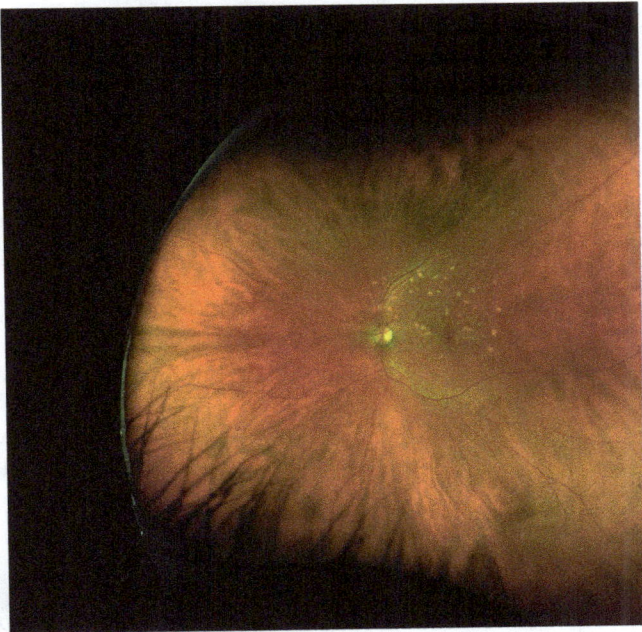

FIGURE 9.5 Butterfly-shaped pigment dystrophy.

macula predominantly and basically can look like a big patch of GA. Technically, there is no clean cutoff between these types; it is more of a spectrum, and whilst it is confusing, it is important to be aware of it.

Lastly, while several of the above subtypes can indeed be *confused with macular degeneration*, we now come to the category (another umbrella as it turns out) of things that can **really** be confused with macular degeneration. Again, there is no real purpose in being able to name all of these conditions like some sort of Rain Man, but it might be useful to know which entities are hiding under this particular umbrella. Sorsby pseudoinflammatory fundus dystrophy looks like aggressive dry macular degeneration, but can cause added confusion, as it is very common as a complication of this for actual neovascular CNVM (not strictly speaking 'macular degeneration') to occur. Malattia Leventinese, also confusingly called familial dominant drusen (probably the preferred term as it is more descriptive) and Doyne honeycomb retinal dystrophy describe aggressive drusen formation, and potential secondary neovascularisation, from an age much younger than with regular macular degeneration. It is, as the name suggests, inherited in a dominant fashion, and whilst the fact that the name implies it is a disease of the Levantine valley somewhere in Switzerland, this is untrue because it is present in many parts of the world. You might have heard of other conditions such as North Carolina macular dystrophy, and whilst there are indeed many other variants that are named and fit into this category, please don't spend time worrying about knowing what they are. Put simply, if an apparent macular degeneration of whatever ilk presents early or oddly, or if there is a family history, then consider an inherited condition.

Christiana Says...

Acquired vitelliform lesions are similar in appearance to adult vitelliform dystrophy but with no clear genetic cause, can be unilateral or bilateral and can be associated with other retinal diseases including age-related macular degeneration (AMD) and central serous chorioretinopathy. Stargardt disease is the most common inherited macular dystrophy and is typically diagnosed in children and teenagers due to mutations in the ABCA4 gene. The ABCA4 gene produces a protein that clears toxic byproducts of vitamin A in photoreceptors. However, I must flag the late-onset Stargardt disease variant: some people develop the disease late because they have milder mutations that reduce the function of the protein as opposed to completely disabling it, which results in earlier onset and more rapid progression. Late-onset Stargardt disease and GA can look similar clinically because both cause progressive central vision loss and atrophy of the macula. Some tips to differentiate them are that you may see flecks that show increased autofluorescence on fundus autofluorescence (FAF), no drusen and less extensive and less confluent choriocapillaris loss on OCT angiography (OCT-A) in Stargardt's disease than GA. This distinction is even more important as we approach selecting patients with GA for treatment.

INVESTIGATIONS

The first investigation, of course, is an OCT scan, which is something usually undertaken before the patient has even been seen by you. Almost always, unless you have some fancy widefield OCT device, this will be a macular OCT alone. With primarily

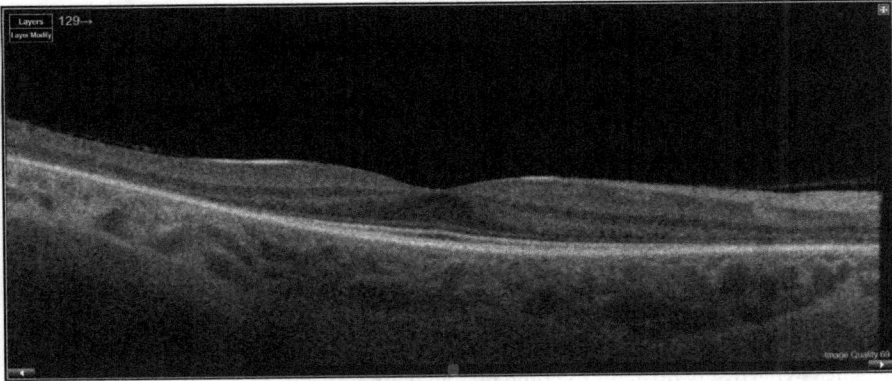

FIGURE 9.6 Thinning of the retina with loss of the ellipsoid zone on an optical coherence tomography (OCT) scan of a patient with RP.

retinal dystrophies, the thing to look for is retinal thinning on the far extremities of the scan with loss of the ellipsoid zone (see Figure 9.6). Obviously, if the condition is advanced, then this will be closer to the fovea, and if it is early, it might not have reached the area of the OCT at all and all will look normal. If it is a macular dystrophy, then appearances can vary from very slight to catastrophically bad, depending on the condition. Either way, look at the RPE and ellipsoid layer for disruption and thinning. Look out for cystoid macular oedema (CMO) as well, as this is a marker of the function of the pumping action of the pigment epithelium.

FAF is a very good mapper of RPE health, revealing black areas of dead RPE along with brighter areas of overfunctioning stressed cells being slowly worked to death. FAF is a good way of mapping progress and therefore working out the prognosis (well, roughly). The other benefit of this is that widefield FAF is far more widespread and therefore easier to access in regular eye units. FAF, along with colour fundus photography, should ideally be performed at each and every appointment, usually a year apart, again, to gauge progress. After all, speed cameras work by taking two pictures separated by a set time to establish speed. Certain lesions rich in lipofuscin such as those found in Stargardt disease also show up really nicely.

In many textbooks, fundus fluorescein angiography (FFA) and indocyanine green angiography (ICGA) results are described in detail for each and every variant of inherited retinal disease, but since those textbooks were written, access to genetic testing has improved, and we are moving away from a phenotypic way of describing variants to a genotypic way, which hopefully at some point will reap some kind of reward via the development of some sort of therapy, though this seems as long away as the practical use of nuclear fusion at present. It is not usual to routinely perform FFA or ICGA in these patients now unless the diagnosis is in doubt, although the images are beautiful and striking and display much loved signs such as a dark choroid, can show accurately the health of the RPE and measure the active leakage that may not be seen so well on the OCT scan. However, unlike the other tests, they carry risks.

Visual field testing can be a way of tracking progress as well as the above tests, with 120 dot full fields being best if the disease is very peripheral, with Humphrey visual fields being possible as the advancing border of doom approaches closer to the back of the eye. An Esterman binocular field is important in determining whether the patient can carry on driving or not.

Electrophysiology is especially important, though most units will have to send their patients to some other institution for the test to be performed. Asking for an electroretinogram (ERG) and pattern electroretinogram (PERG) is the minimum, though usually sensible electophysiologists will perform more tests depending on the diagnosis you're querying, whether you've asked for them or not. Best disease, for example, needs an electrooculogram (EOG). In Wales, there is only one health board that has the full suite of ophthalmic electrophysiology tests at its disposal, mainly because expertise is difficult to come by and economies of scale are needed to properly administer this valuable asset. Not just anyone can do it; well, at least do it well. Despite all our reading for the Fellowship of the Royal College of Ophthalmologists (FRCOphth) exam, unless you have a special interest or work in a very large centre, you won't really understand the A waves and B waves and what the values and deviations mean. It really is purposeless to pretend that you do. Nobody's fooled. What pretty much everyone does is look straight at the report at the end of all the fancy graphs and lines and then perhaps in a bit of theatre in front of the patient, ponder the traces for a few seconds for effect before deciding that the report is in fact correct and you agree with the findings.

For practical purposes, the electrophysiology report will say what the rod function is, what the cone function is, the general function and will have a component for special tests undertaken such as an EOG. Good reports will tell you if the test results fit the diagnosis on the form, and if not, what other differential diagnoses could account for the findings observed. This could well be considered the last test needed before referring the patient for the definitive test, the genetic test itself.

Whilst in theory anyone can order genetic tests, in fact, anyone ordering them is not generally good. An infrastructure is needed of genetic counselling, support for various diagnoses, access to research trials, and knowledge of the different gene panels that exist in your local area or nationally is all sacrosanct. If you don't have all of these things, then it's not good simply winging it and trying to do it yourself. These tests have consequences and research-wise it is essential that clinicians that are plugged into all the latest trials, ideally professors and academics, manage these patients. However, their precious time is limited and that is why we need to first discern very roughly that there is something going on and have a stab at what that might, in fact, be. ERG and PERG evidence of some kind of dysfunction is essential really; you don't want to refer normal patients, glaucoma patients or other non-genetic patients to them. It's okay if your diagnosis is wrong; the genetic test is the ultimate powerful arbiter and will correct any misunderstanding along the way.

Christiana Says...

On the subject of trials, Tinlarebant is an investigational drug being evaluated for Stargardt disease. It is an oral small molecule inhibitor of retinol-binding protein 4 (RBP4) that reduces the delivery of vitamin A to the retina by inhibiting RBP4. This lowers the formation of toxic vitamin A byproducts that cause damage to the RPE and photoreceptors in Stargardt disease. This treatment is currently in phase 3 trial (the DRAGON study) and has recently been granted breakthrough therapy designation by the U.S. Food and Drug Administration (FDA), which expedites development and review when preliminary evidence suggests the drug may demonstrate substantial improvement compared to standard of care.

MANAGEMENT

We have covered management above insofar as suspecting the patient has a genetic condition and undertaking the appropriate investigations in the right order is concerned. Obtaining a full and comprehensive family history is also essential if any other members have any eye conditions of a similar nature. It is useful to draw these relationships in the notes using the square and circle family tree diagrams so beloved amongst clinical geneticists. Our role essentially as non-experts in these very complex conditions is to recognise the potential for a genetic condition, and send the patient to the appropriate expert for genetic testing. We then get a response letter (usually many, many months later) saying the gene panel showed some mutations, which they will then name, and which we will not usually understand. It will be a combination of letters and numbers, but it will say if it is either a dominant, recessive, X-linked or sporadic condition, or whether nothing unusual was found at all. Usually, they would have had this explained to them at far greater length and detail by the good professor than we would ever have been able to do.

Our role is to follow up locally as needed, usually once a year will suffice, offering support of various hues. This support is indeed important and consists of offering a certificate of visual impairment (CVI), either as sight impaired or severely sight impaired, when the criteria are met. This should be done with input from the eye clinic liaison officer along with support from charitable organisations such as the Royal National Institute for the Blind (RNIB) and the macular society for example, though there are myriad charities depending on what the exact condition turns out to be. Having a steady supply of leaflets and access to support is very important, as patients will forget much of what you say to them during the consultation itself. Do not underestimate the importance this follow-up every year or so has on the patient and their family, or even yourself and your team. As you see them grow and change, and you measure rates of deterioration and discuss the future with them, you perform more of the work of an old-fashioned Hippocratic doctor than anyone really performs in the modern world now. We learn a lot ourselves.

From a medical standpoint, a check every year also allows for complications to be found and sorted out. Of these, there are two main things to watch out for; the development of cataracts and the development of CMO. Patients with inherited retinal dystrophies tend to develop posterior subcapsular cataracts at a much earlier age than the general population, and it is important to watch out for this, as cataract surgery is the only practical thing we can do that actually has a chance to improve sight. Should a patient complain of a sudden and unexpected deterioration in vision 1 year to the next, think of cataract in the first instance and have a low threshold for listing for surgery. Do not listen to those who might try to rationalise that cataract surgery would produce lower benefits than in patients unaffected by a genetic condition and as such is not in their best interests due to the cost–benefit ratio. They are wrong.

The development of CMO over time is as a result of increasing dysfunction of the RPE cells, and as such, the fluid is totally immune to any anti-vascular endothelial growth factor (anti-VEGF) or steroid injection. Many inherited conditions mentioned above are, in fact, associated with the development of secondary CNVM development, though here the OCT characteristics and history will be different, more sudden and depending on the location, more visually disabling, with the presence of blood making the nature of the lesion much more obvious to the clinician. It is therefore important to tell these two entities apart, and Chapter 5 will assist the reader in this. CMO associated with RPE dysfunction in inherited conditions is usually mild, less visually disabling and bilateral, though it can be asymmetrical.

Treating this fluid is tricky. The only real way that this can be approached with even a slight chance of some success is through carbonic anhydrase inhibitors. These are usually used in glaucoma and derive their function here through their effect on the RPE cells' pumping action; in the way that riot police entering a striking mine might try to operate some of the machinery themselves to get some coal moving at least. As with the mine analogy, these medications are only very partially successful, if they have any effect at all, although there are unusual cases where the effect is profound. The classic medication that is used is dorzolamide (Trusopt) three times daily, though sometimes oral acetazolamide 250 mg twice daily is used instead. However, this is generally frowned upon due to the increased side effects and complications that can occur, whereas instilling drops is usually no great bother. The key is working out if the drops do anything. If, on follow-up, say, 3 months after the medication has been commenced, OCT scanning does indicate that the fluid has reduced in volume and the patient has noticed the benefit, then continuing would be the best course of action. If the patient has not noticed any improvement, either subjectively or objectively, then there is little purpose in continuing.

Sometimes patients will ask you to examine family members who happen to come with them for any signs of the same condition. Do not, under any circumstances, be tempted to do a quick ad hoc examination in clinic to look for basic signs, with an undiluted eye and without having the time to take a proper history or do any of the proper tests. Ask the patient to have their relative referred in the proper manner so that everything can be done properly, if there are symptoms, or examined by a qualified optometrist for signs in case referral is needed if not. Anything short of this will store up trouble for the future.

Christiana Says...

Carbonic anhydrase inhibitors reduce the production of aqueous humour and may also improve fluid resorption at the RPE by altering PH and ionic gradients, helping reduce cystoid spaces. There are many small open-label and randomised controlled studies demonstrating reduction in central macular thickness and modest improvement in visual acuity in some patients treated with topical dorzolamide and oral acetazolamide (1). However, there are no large, controlled studies, and therefore these treatments are off-label. Treatment usually starts with topical carbonic anhydrase due to the better safety profile, and if there is insufficient response, oral acetazolamide is considered. Some authors have explored the use of intravitreal anti-VEGF in these cases, with demonstrable anatomical response but no improvement in visual acuity. These agents are consequently not recommended for CMO secondary to retinal dystrophies.

THE FUTURE

Patients sometimes bring in newspaper clippings from notorious sources with hopeful articles about some breakthrough or other that has been made somewhere. These articles are morally reprehensible on multiple fronts; there is an unholy alliance of researchers, many fellow ophthalmologists, pushing the narrative hard to overstate the importance of their work to get more funding with the newspapers who know the truth full well taking advantage of this to sell more papers. At the end of the day, patients are then misled into thinking that they need not fear too much for the future, as a cure is at hand. It is not, and this cruel practice must end!

If anyone mentions developments in gene therapy or stem cell research to you, it is best to have a sympathetic spiel prepared that will reverse engineer these expectations in a gentle, humanistic way. Very occasionally, patients will try to raise money for trips to China or Russia for untried, untested experimental therapies that have been sold to them by snake oil salesmen online, backed up by papers written in journals you've never heard of purporting success. Never support these trips, and never lend even a modicum of support to such fundraising activities. The world is a dark place where evil people take advantage of the fact that no treatment exists for these conditions affecting innocent young people, and it is up to us to be their protectors and guardians.

REFERENCE

1. Huang Q, Chen R, Lin X, Xiang Z. Efficacy of carbonic anhydrase inhibitors in management of cystoid macular edema in retinitis pigmentosa: A meta-analysis. PLoS One. 2017; 12(10):e0186180. doi: 10.1371/journal.pone.0186180.

10 Other Important Medical Retina Conditions

We have covered many important diagnoses in medical retina, and by volume, work that will perhaps account for more than 95% of all the medical retina patients that we will see. Neovascular age-related macular degeneration (nAMD) and diabetic eye disease alone will account for absolutely staggering patient numbers, clinic time and departmental resources. But there are other diseases in the world of medical retina that we come across, without knowledge of which we would not be fully qualified all round practitioners in the glorious field of Medical Retina. We will now explore these conditions in turn in a practical, sensible way.

MACULAR TELANGIECTASIA

There are two subsets of this condition that you will come across, handily called Type 1 and Type 2. Type 1 macular telangiectasia, often referred to by the shorter, jazzier MacTel title, is, in a nutshell, when some sort of malformation of the capillary network temporal to the fovea causes an exudative leakage. It has been compared to a macular subset of Coat's disease (see below). Patients are younger than with any condition that might form a differential diagnosis such as a branch retinal vein occlusion (BRVO), and optical coherence tomography (OCT) scanning reveals a hefty amount of intraretinal fluid present. OCT angiography (OCT-A) can reveal the telangiectatic vessels and aneurysms nicely under ideal circumstances, but it is fundus fluorescein angiography (FFA) that really identifies Type 1 MacTel for what it is. Treatment, if required, is with either an intravitreal Ozurdex injection or focal laser, though these have significantly variable results. Anti-vascular endothelial growth factor (anti-VEGF) injections generally do much less, and most other things do nothing at all.

Type 2 MacTel is confusing because it is really nothing at all like Type 1. It is bilateral for a start, whereas Type 1 is almost always unilateral. There is no exudation either. The macular area generally collapses in on itself, leaving structural voids that can sometimes be mistaken for fluid, and well, technically it is, but it is not leaking; it simply exists in spaces because the retina has died around it. It can be mistaken for macular degeneration, although the OCT scan involves the whole retinal thickness (see Figure 10.1). Confusingly, as with any destructive retinal process, a secondary choroidal neovascular membrane (CNVM) can grow through this scar and cause a true exudative leakage. The reason this develops is unknown. There are several hypotheses, including nutrition and such, but it's all guesswork, really. There is no treatment at all that exists for the process itself at present.

Christiana Says...

MacTel Type 2 is an idiopathic disease, typically presenting in the 4th to 6th decade, with a prevalence of 0.004% to 0.1%. It appears to be a primary neurodegenerative

DOI: 10.1201/9781003628309-10

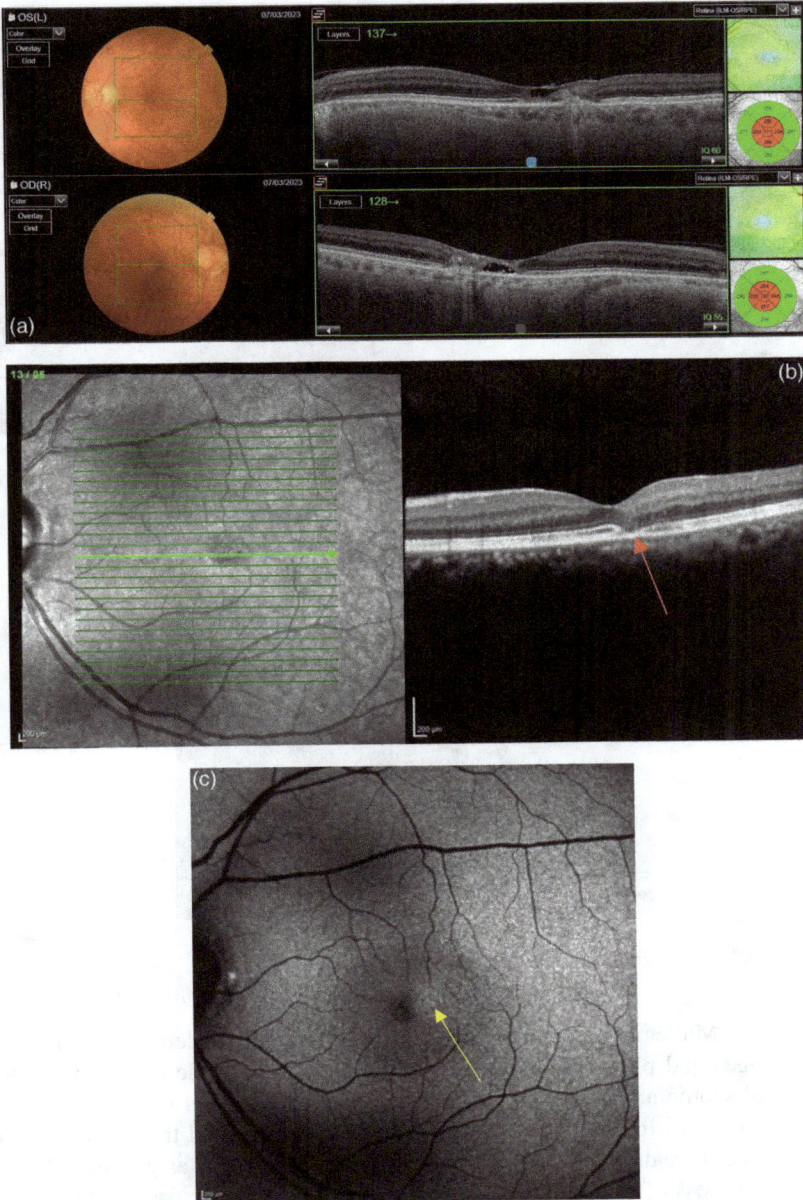

FIGURE 10.1   (a) An optical coherence tomography (OCT) scan of a patient with Type 2 macular telangiectasia (MacTel). (b) OCT in early MacTel Type 2. Red arrow denotes disruption of the ellipsoid zone temporal to the fovea. (c) Fundus autofluorescence (FAF) in early MacTel Type 2. Yellow arrow denotes increased autofluorescence temporal to the fovea. (d) OCT in late MacTel Type 2. FAF in late MacTel Type 2 (6 years later). Red arrow denotes pigment migration. Yellow arrow denotes extended ellipsoid zone disruption. (e) FAF 6 years later. Red arrow denotes pigment hyperpigmentation that blocks autofluorescence. *(Continued)*

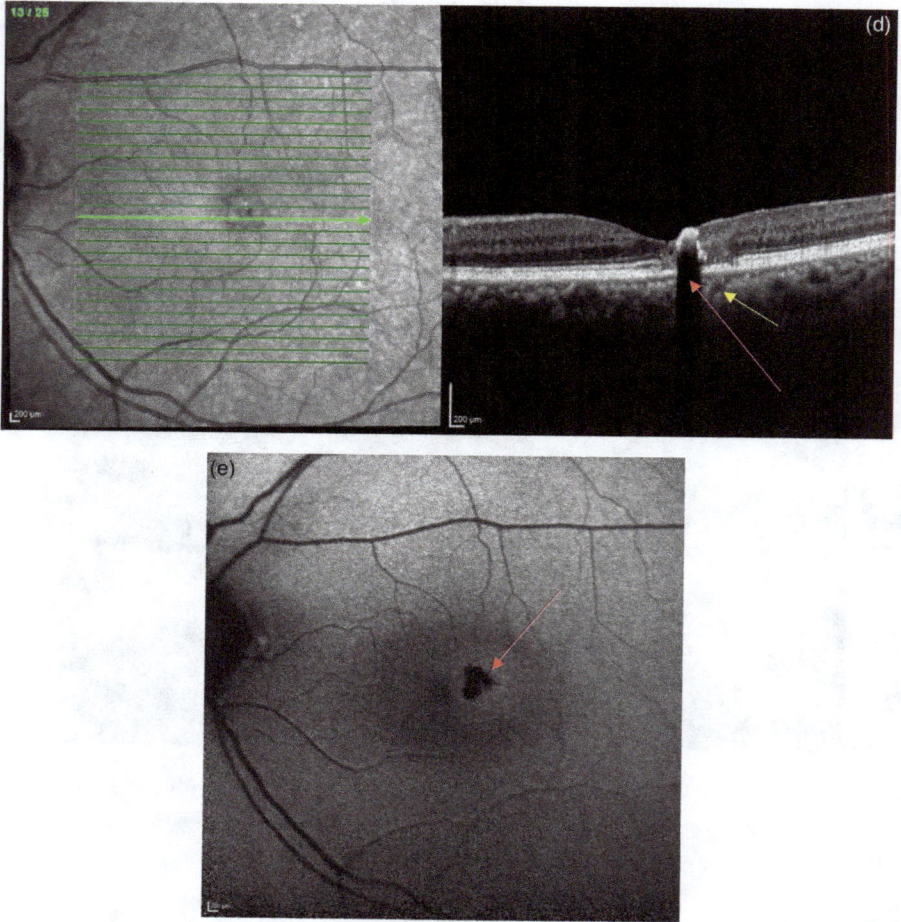

FIGURE 10.1 *(Continued)*

disease, with Muller cell dysfunction and macular pigment depletion preceding vascular changes and photoreceptor loss. Early symptoms include difficulty reading, paracentral scotoma and metamorphopsia. Distortion becomes more prominent as the fovea becomes involved. Early signs include loss of retinal transparency in the temporal juxtafoveal region, which can be seen on fundoscopy as greying. On FAF, there is early loss of hypoautofluorescence at the fovea due to loss of macular pigment. As the disease progresses, OCT reveals inner retinal cavitations or spaces, retinal thinning and ellipsoid zone disruption, particularly temporal to the fovea and pigment hyperplasia (see Table 10.1).

Visual prognosis is variable, though legal blindness rarely occurs in the context of extensive atrophy. In March 2025, the U.S. Food and Drug Administration (FDA) approved Encelto, a small intravitreous implant, inserted through a small scleral incision. It contains allogeneic retinal pigment epithelial cells engineered to

TABLE 10.1

Features of Type 2 Macular Telangiectasia

Features of MacTel Type 2

Early

Loss of retinal transparency in the temporal juxtafoveal region

Right angled venules

Retinal telangiectasia, mainly temporal to fovea

Loss of hypoautofluorescence at the fovea on FAF

Later

Inner retinal cavitations on OCT

Crystalline deposits in the inner retina

Retinal thinning on OCT

Disruption of ellipsoid zone on OCT

continuously secrete ciliary neurotropic factor (CNTF). CNTF has been shown to slow the progression of MacTel Type 2 (1).

COATS DISEASE AND COATS-LIKE RETINOPATHY

These two conditions are clinically pretty much the same but present in different age groups. Coats, of course, is the original and described a progressive developmental abnormality of peripheral blood vessels, almost always in one eye of usually male children. There is an association with various genetic disorders such as facioscapulohumeral dystrophy and Turner syndrome. There is telangiectasia and aneurysms with increasing amounts of exudation that can spread centrally and not only threaten but overwhelm the fovea. There is also capillary dropout and increasing areas of peripheral ischaemia that develop over time. It usually isn't seen by proper Medical Retina specialists, mainly because it is almost always dealt with by our paediatric brethren before the patient comes of age to be seen by us. Diagnosis is by and large with a widefield FFA, although OCT may come into play if the macula is threatened.

Treatment is generally dependent on how bad it is; if it is mild and off in the periphery, then it can be documented by photography and watched, but if it worsens, then after mapping with FFA, the affected areas can be lasered with panretinal photocoagulation (PRP) in a low-power, long-duration manner ('low and slow') to control the leakage. If the exudation becomes too bad for laser to touch, then cryotherapy can be used, but if this battle is lost again and the retina becomes detached through exudation, then our vitreoretinal colleagues may need to be contacted to perform surgery to drain fluid. Sometimes this battle too is lost, and a blind eye becomes a painful blind eye with the retina floating up to touch the lens itself with subsequent pressure issues that only an evisceration/enucleation can solve. Treatment with anti-VEGF doesn't really do anything, and though Ozurdex can work, it is a holding action more than anything else. There are many different grading systems, though these are useless and redundant in the modern era of widefield photography, when even the minutest of changes can be tracked, though the Puritans will, of course, deny this.

Coats disease is interesting, and although it doesn't really involve us, it is true is that the older the presentation of the patient in general, the more positive the prognosis and less aggressive the disease. If this condition appears in adulthood, especially older adults, it is referred to as Coats-like retinopathy instead. The naming can be confusing because there are multiple names for things here, as with many frustrating areas of medical retina. Lebers miliary aneurysms is another name for Coats, whereas Coats-like exudative vitreoretinopathy and similar variants are alternatives for Coats-like. In truth, there isn't a proper cutoff between Coats and Coats-like except age and aggression, though you could argue that diminishing aggression with age is a feature of Coats anyway, so it's just an extension of that. As mentioned above, Type 1 MacTel is considered by some to be another sort of variant of this whole telangiectatic aneurysmal exudative spectrum.

We will indeed come across Coats-like retinopathy, though the treatment and management are much the same; monitoring with Optos photography, with widefield FFA if the condition deteriorates so that sectoral retinal laser can be planned (low and slow). Should the condition continue to deteriorate despite this, we involve our vitreoretinal friends so that cryo can be performed, or surgery proper if the retina floats off. By and large, the whole thing is a lot less aggressive though, and therefore it can be argued that Ozurdex has a slightly bigger role than in children, especially in flattening things so that retinal laser can be made more effective.

CHOROIDAL NAEVI AND MELANOMAS

One of the great curses, as well as the boons, of recent developments in primary care eye services has been the increased availability of fundus photography. Members of the European race, especially northern Europeans and Celts, have freckles. We are freckly naevic people. Almost one in ten of us similarly have choroidal naevi, but as we typically cannot see within our own eyeball, it falls to an ever eager optometrist to see a naevus and then panic both the patient and the hospital by sending in an urgent referral detailing what they say is a 'new' finding, though in fact it may just be the first time that patient has been photographed by anyone.

There are many different ways of assessing these naevi, but the MOLES system is a good one. Table 10.2 demonstrates how a choroidal naevus is scored under this

TABLE 10.2
The MOLES Scoring System

MOLES Signs	Score
Mushroom shape	Absent = 0, Erosion through RPE but indistinct = 1, Present = 2
Orange pigment	Absent = 0, Dusting = 1, Confluent, easily visible = 2
Large size	Flat or <1 mm thick and less than 3 disc diameters wide = 0, 1 – 2mm thick and/or 3–4 disc diameters wide = 1, >2 mm thick and/or >4 disc diameters wide = 2
Enlargement	None = 0, Suspected change = 1, Definite change = 2
Subretinal fluid	Nil = 0, Trace, seen only on OCT = 1, Define, seen on fundoscopy = 2

system, which is an acronym standing for five different important things to look out for.

If the total score is a happy zero, then the patient needn't have been referred to you in the first place, and they can be discharged back to the optometrist for routine follow-up, or ideally retained in the community in the first place. If the score is 1 or 2, then a non-urgent referral to the hospital is recommended, and some sort of virtual pigmented naevi system is ideal for dealing with this sort of thing in which trained staff performing widefield photography, OCT and B-scan ultrasound can separate the wheat from the chaff (and there is an awful lot of chaff). If after 2 or 3 yearly visits everything seems stable, then depending on your optometric partner, these patients can again be discharged to the community or followed up in the hospital if the necessary expertise there is lacking. Only if the MOLES score is 3 or more can an urgent referral to your medical retina clinic be justified and the case treated as urgent suspected cancer (USC) with its 2-week referral to assessment time.

Our role when we see these patients face-to-face is to confirm the MOLES score and ask about symptoms, family history, past medical history and such. If we have a wide open door for naevi in view of their sheer numbers we will be inundated, so it is sacrosanct that we only open it for those who truly need to see us. Our roles then, as general Medical Retina specialists not working in an ocular oncology centre of excellence, is to work out what to send on to the great and the good at Moorfields, Liverpool or the other big United Kingdom oncology units. In the same way that we don't want to be inundated by chaff, neither should we want to inundate our onco-logical colleagues. Only refer cases that are truly suspicious of melanoma.

It is not for us to discuss here how these lesions should be treated by an ocular oncology centre, except to say very generally that they either write back asking us to monitor the patient, undertake ruthenium plaque brachytherapy, or perform some other sort of treatment. The experts then send the patient back to us and ask us to see them every so often, though they rarely say for how long, so we end up seeing them every year or so forever, being too scared to discharge them and too timid to write and ask the simple question 'for how long?' Funnily enough, when we do ask, the answer is rarely simple or straightforward and usually amounts to some vague instruction that we dutifully file in the notes but don't understand.

One of the complications that results from radiation is radiation retinopathy, which can lead to cystoid macular oedema (CMO). The treatment for this is a treat-and-extend anti-VEGF regimen that again might well carry on forever. Occasionally, the oncology team will write back saying an enucleation is needed but that the patient has 'opted to have this done locally'. If this is the case, a friendly letter to our oculoplastic colleagues will do the trick. Otherwise, our role is to perform widefield photography once a year, comparing pictures, and checking for cataract, fluid and answering questions.

Christiana Says...

Radiation retinopathy is an unfortunate consequence of treatment often delivered to save sight or indeed life (nasopharyngeal tumours, for example). It is a chronic, progressive occlusive vasculopathy resulting from ionizing radiation exposure. Clinical onset often occurs 6 months to 3 years post-treatment, though this can vary. Radiation causes damage to the endothelial cells, leading to capillary non-perfusion, ischaemia, VEGF upregulation and progressive vascular leakage. Systemic conditions that cause endothelial cell dysfunction, such as diabetes and hypertension amplify the risk of radiation retinopathy. Clinically, the features are similar to diabetic retinopathy, with microaneurysm, telangiectasias, cotton wool spots and retinal haemorrhages. Anti-VEGF therapy is the mainstay of treatment, often requiring frequent dosing, but other treatment modalities such as intravitreal steroids and laser have been tried with varying results in refractory cases.

CONGENITAL HYPERTROPHY OF THE RETINAL PIGMENT EPITHELIUM

A hamartoma is defined as a benign malformation of cells that are normally found in the tissue in question. The most common retinal hamartoma is congenital hypertrophy of the retinal pigment epithelium (CHRPE) in which, as the name suggests, there is an abnormal overgrowth of retinal pigment epithelium (RPE) cells. They are not naevi. CHRPE can present in three flavours: solitary, grouped or atypical.

Solitary CHRPE lesions consist of a single patch of uniformly darkened (grey to jet black) patch of retina with a sharply demarcated edge, which might be surrounded by a thin halo of depigmentation. Sometimes there are round, well-demarcated holes of depigmentation within the lesion, which are termed lacunae. Figure 10.2 illustrates a typical solitary CHRPE lesion. It is of no consequence at all, except that occasionally it can cause confusion, with some people mistaking it for a naevus or

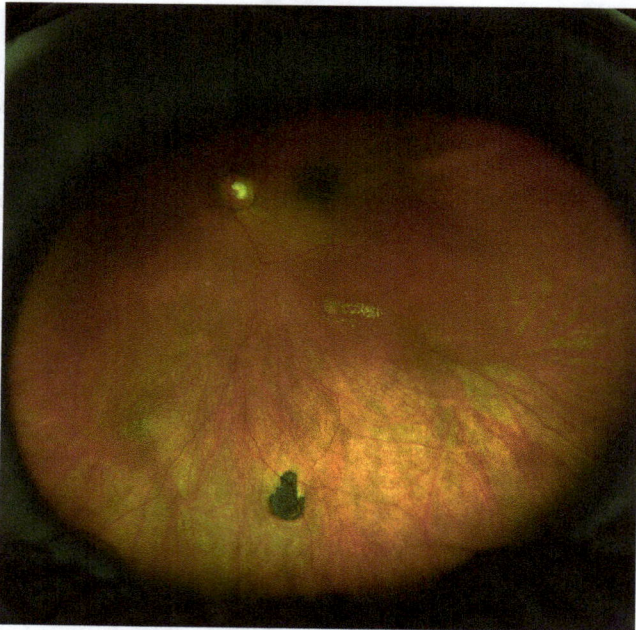

FIGURE 10.2 A solitary CHRPE lesion.

even a melanoma. The patient simply needs to be reassured and a picture taken for the records.

Grouped CHRPE lesions are commonly called 'bear track' lesions because although these well-demarcated spots of hyperpigmentation are indeed grouped, they tend to be in two or three clusters of smaller lesions that do sort of resemble the paw prints of some large animal that has ambled across the retina at some point. Sometimes these look white and are quite cutely called polar bear tracks in that situation. Again, the only treatment is picture taking, reassurance and discharge back to their optometrist.

Atypical CHRPE lesions are again multiple, though instead of being grouped in nice clusters, might be haphazardly distributed throughout the fundus of one, or more commonly both, eyes. These lesions tend to be oval- or spindle-shaped and classically described as 'pisciform' as they can look like fish. This is mainly associated with familial adenomatous polyposis coli, also called Gardner's syndrome, where the same genetic defect that causes this issue in the eye, which does not cause any serious issue in itself at that location, is associated with the growth of multiple cancerous polyps in the bowel. This is not an uncommon exam question, and many eyecare professionals are very aware of this, but in reality you won't see any fresh new case in your life in which the bowel issue is unknown until you've skillfully suggested a colonoscopy based on your Dr. House examination of the eye. It just won't happen. What will, in fact, happen, is that you will get multiple referrals over your career from clinicians who see perhaps grouped CHRPE, and as they vaguely remember some bowel connection, refer to you to check it out.

ASTROCYTOMA

Retinal astrocytomas are hamartomas as well, though of the glial cells in the nerve fibre layer as opposed to the RPE. There is a dome-shaped whitish lump in the retina that may or may not be multinodular in nature. If they are multinodular, they are sometimes referred to as 'mulberry lesions' after the appearance of the mulberry fruit, though very few of us in this day and age when we hear the name 'mulberry' can actually picture what a mulberry looks like. Retinal astrocytomas are famously associated with a condition called tuberous sclerosis, the classical triad of which consists of epilepsy, mental retardation and skin growths called adenoma sebaceum. In reality, of course, few patients will have this triad, and so a long and complicated diagnostic system exists for tuberous sclerosis based on the presence or absence of multiple signs and symptoms across the whole body.

Despite what you may be told in the large textbooks of ophthalmology, a regular Medical Retina specialist does not need to know how to diagnose tuberous sclerosis. You will never ever find a case of undiagnosed tuberous sclerosis in your clinic through the presence of a retinal astrocytoma. Never. You might be referred a case of suspected tuberous sclerosis and asked to look at the eyes to see if you see any astrocytomas to help other cleverer physicians build a diagnostic case, but more commonly you will find them by chance. Though they are also associated with retinitis pigmentosa, Type 1 neurofibromatosis and Stargardt disease, most of those you will come across will be sporadic and of no clinical consequence. They are

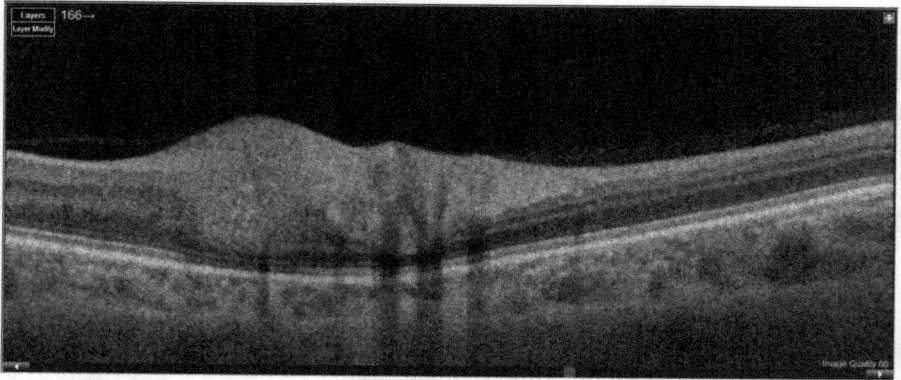

FIGURE 10.3   An OCT scan of a retinal astrocytoma.

asymptomatic, and OCT is the best modality for ensuring your diagnosis is correct mainly because it confirms that the mass is in the nerve fibre layer, with the presence of Swiss cheese holes (as with CHRPE peculiarly) being typical. Figure 10.3 illustrates the OCT appearance of a retinal astrocytoma. Again, the treatment is picture, reassurance and discharge.

COMBINED HAMARTOMA OF THE RETINA AND RPE

Sticking with the theme of hamartomas, the combined hamartoma of the retina and RPE is due to a malformation of not just the RPE as in CHRPE but the whole retina as well. The normal appearance is a pigmented, poorly circumscribed lesion that can have associated vascular abnormalities along with an epiretinal membrane and tractional elements. They tend to be located around the optic disc or macula but can also be more peripheral. Ironically, although the peripheral version is rarer than the posterior pole version, it is the most likely to be found and diagnosed by us, as the more posterior types tend to cause visual issues in childhood and are therefore found by our paediatric ophthalmology colleagues. The appearance can be very variable, but OCT confirms that the retina and RPE are both involved. Although as with all hamartomas, there is nothing much to worry about here from the lesion itself, at least in adulthood when it can't cause amblyopia, confusion can arise when it is mistaken for a more sinister lesion, and there have been cases where eyes have been enucleated in the past in the belief that a melanoma was present. If this is suspected, the patient is of young age, and there is a tractional gliotic element along with pigmentation, then monitoring over a few 6-monthly visits is wise (with pictures, of course) then reassurance and discharge.

RETINAL HAEMANGIOMAS – CAPILLARY, CAVERNOUS AND CHOROIDAL

In yet another hamartomatous maldevelopment, **retinal capillary haemangiomas** are of two varieties: the ones located next to the optic disc that tend to look like a confused reddish pink mess of leakage and hard exudates where the blood vessels are not immediately obvious, and 'proper' peripheral ones not at the disc. The disc variety can mimic disc oedema in younger patients and peripapillary choroidal neo-vascularisation in older patients. The non-juxtapapillary type is easier to spot for what it is, as they are located at the inner retina as opposed to the outer retina and classically have a tortuous feeding artery that is obvious, a swollen haemangioma that is easy to see along with signs of leakage and exudation, as well as a tortuous swollen draining vein. In diagnosing capillary haemangiomas, the peripheral version can be detected clinically, though the more confusing peripapillary version does well with an FFA because the dye highlights the vessels that are otherwise unseen and confirms the peripapillary as opposed to papillary nature of the lesion. OCT doesn't have a role in diagnosis as such, as it just looks like a leaky confused waterlogged retina or disc, but does have a role in monitoring severity, risk to the macula and response to treatment.

There are two things to bear in mind with capillary haemangiomas: why they occurred and what to do about them. The thing that people remember from exams is the association with Von Hippel–Lindau (VHL) syndrome and that this can have angiomas intracranially as well as renal cell tumours and pheochromocytomas. Thankfully, most patients come to us having been diagnosed by the genetics team, and we are asked to monitor the patient's eyes every year or so for the development of capillary haemangioma, which we do gladly in clinic as the visits are usually quick, and the patients get to know us and we save some time in our lives during a busy clinic as most of the time there is nothing new to see.

Sometimes, however, we will be the first to come across a retinal capillary hae-mangioma. Should this happen, don't panic; ask about symptoms of headache and other bodily ills and ask the clinic nurse to take the blood pressure. If the blood pressure is high and symptoms are present, say more than 200/100, then immedi-ate referral to the inpatient medical team is needed in case a pheochromocytoma is present, but this is thankfully rarely the case. Usually, the blood pressure is fine and there are no symptoms of anything. In this case, if only one haemangioma has been found (and one is enough for anyone), then a tentative computerized tomog-raphy (CT) angiogram can be ordered to look for intracranial abnormalities, and if none are found, we can cautiously say it is unrelated to VHL and concentrate on the haemangioma alone. If there is more than one, then immediate referral to a clinical geneticist is warranted, as they are best placed to know what all the latest diagnostic procedures are, to sort out counselling and so on; the rest of the body is no place for an ophthalmologist. Should there be only one, but the CT reveals an intracranial vas-cular anomaly, then we can refer at that point. We should, under no circumstances, order magnetic resonance imaging (MRI) of the abdomen or urine tests for vanillyl-mandelic acid. We just become suspicious and send the patient to people who know what they are doing.

From a treatment perspective regarding the eye, try to do as much masterly inac-tivity as possible. Watch and wait and wait and watch. Take pictures and compare. If the vision is not threatened and the lesion is off to the side, just watch it every few weeks or months at increasing intervals until you're satisfied it's not doing anything evil. If the peripheral version's leakage starts threatening the macula and vision, then argon laser is the first port of call. Surrounding the haemangioma with burns while

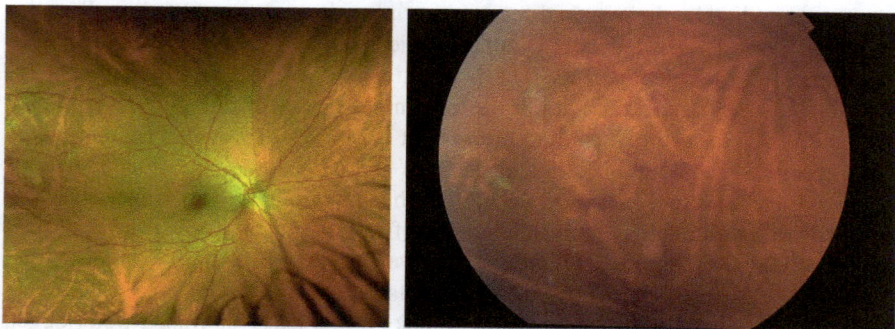

FIGURE 10.4   The key features of a capillary haemangioma.

also hitting the feeder vessel over several sessions, followed by hitting the mass itself, can shut it down. Don't hit the mass until you've stopped the artery, or massive bleeding will take place. Similarly, don't hit the vein. If this doesn't work, ask your friendly local vitreoretinal surgeons if they can perform cryotherapy. Should this also not work, then don't keep hitting it with more of the same; refer to an ocular oncology unit for more powerful treatments such as radiotherapy. The peripapillary version is much more difficult to treat properly because it is next to the disc, which can hold it hostage. In this eventuality, photodynamic therapy is the best bet, but this too might be best undertaken by an ocular oncology unit. Figure 10.4 illustrates the key features of a capillary haemangioma.

A **cavernous retinal haemangioma** can be thought of as dilated grape-like balloons of blood on the inner retina surface, mixed with whitish bands and plaques of gliosis. They can be anywhere on the retina, can be of variable size, and generally don't have an obvious and vibrant connection to the ocular circulation. The diagnosis is clinical, though OCT scanning is useful for confirming the nature of the haemangioma and an FFA, if needed, confirms the lack of a significant blood flow. There is no VHL equivalent here of a distinct condition that can cause this, but there is an association with intracranial cavernous haemangiomas, which can cause death, and so a CT angiogram or MRI equivalent, as with retinal capillary haemangiomas, is a must. If this is normal, then we can settle back and deal only with the eye, but if something is found, then we need to urgently refer the patient to a neurosurgeon. Regarding the retinal lesion, the best delivery of medical care is to do as much nothing as possible, to quote Samuel Shem, and this is true here as well. Take pictures and monitor, but try to refrain from doing anything. Over time, the gliotic bands increase as the blood-filled portions decrease, and we can all breathe a sigh of relief. If they bleed into the vitreous, then a vitreoretinal surgeon's assistance might be sought. It is only very rarely that we are called upon to laser the lesions but if we are, as with their capillary cousins, surround them first before lasering the lesions themselves, but honestly, try to avoid doing this if you can. Figure 10.5 illustrates how a cavernous haemangioma, after bleeding and thus generating a gliotic reaction, can become very difficult to distinguish from other scarring pathologies in the eye.

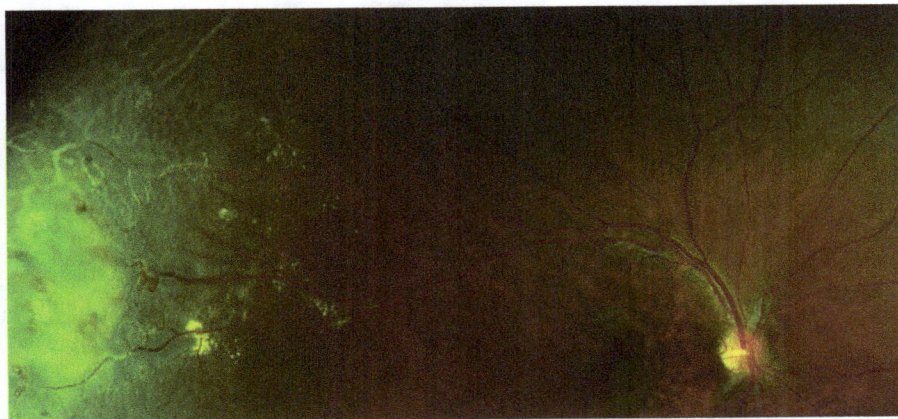

FIGURE 10.5   A cavernous haemangioma in the gliotic phase.

A **racemose haemangioma** isn't a haemangioma and therefore has an annoying name. It is a congenital retinal arteriovenous malformation that is associated with impressively dilated wide-bore vessels in the retina, but usually doesn't leak or cause eye problems as such. Again, it can be associated with intracranial arteriovenous abnormalities, and if so, is called Wyburn–Mason syndrome. It is usually the paediatric ophthalmologist that sees it, but should it be you in your general medical retina clinic, you've guessed it, perform neuroimaging to look at the intracranial blood vessels.

If the choroid is the location of the haemangioma, a **choroidal haemangioma**, then it can be more difficult to detect. This is mainly because we see the bulging retina, but there are no signs of abnormal vessels that we see with the other types discussed thus far. There are two types: a circumscribed choroidal haemangioma and a diffuse type. As the name suggests, the circumscribed type is round and dome-like and has a well-defined border that can be seen on examination, but especially on OCT scanning, which can also demonstrate the presence and extent of subretinal fluid (the main cause of angst). The main differential to watch out for here is choroidal metastases or amelanotic melanoma. B-scan ultrasound is good for separating a choroidal melanoma from the others because it has high internal reflectivity, the same as the surrounding tissue really, as opposed to others that have low internal reflectivity. OCT scanning may also reveal, should you have access to the expensive versions that can see deeply such as enhanced-depth imaging (EDI), enlarged vascular spaces in the choroid and confirms the gentle dome shape so characteristic. The ultimate arbiter, however, is FFA and indocyanine green angiography (ICGA), which reveal rapid filling of the space, as would be expected, whereas any other sort of lesion such as a metastasis or a melanoma, on account of the cellular non-vascular nature of those lesions, do not demonstrate this characteristic.

There is no systemic abnormality associated with this circumscribed type of haemangioma, though for the diffuse variety, this is not true. This type is, as the name suggests, not well circumscribed, does not have an obvious dome-like border, and is said to have a distinctive tomato-ketchup–coloured fundal appearance. This variety is more likely to be associated with systemic conditions such as Sturge–Weber syndrome (SWS). SWS consists of a triad of port wine stain on the face (the same lesion the last Soviet premiere Mikhail Gorbachev had on his baldpate), meningeal capillary-venous malformations and the diffuse choroidal haemangiomas discussed above. For this reason, it will almost always be the case that we will be asked by paediatricians to look into the eyes to see if a diffuse choroidal haemangioma is present. It is an impossibly rare probability indeed that you, as a Medical Retina specialist, will find a diffuse choroidal haemangioma in a patient with a port wine stain and wonder if SWS is present, deciding to perform neuroimaging to look for the third aspect of the triad.

From an ophthalmic perspective, the only thing to think about is the amount of subretinal fluid present and whether it is threatening the macula. If there is increasing fluid present and the visual acuity is falling, then a referral to an ocular oncology centre for photodynamic therapy is indicated. After this, which usually works quite well, the patient is sent back to us, and we simply monitor every 5 or 12 months or so, referring the patient back for more PDT should the fluid return. Sometimes radiotherapy or some other treatment is indicated, but this is not for us simple folk to worry about; our duty is simply to recognise when treatment is needed and to refer to the experts.

VASOPROLIFERATIVE TUMOURS

Despite the scary-sounding name, these lesions are benign. Unlike the hamartomas mentioned above, this is thought to be a form of abnormal healing reaction that sometimes occurs sporadically, but is more commonly related to some kind of ocular pathology such as uveitis, trauma or retinitis pigmentosa. They consist of a growth of local vasculature as well as glial cells and tend to occur (thankfully) in the periphery rather than the posterior pole. Clinically, they look a lot like capillary haemangiomas in that they have a vascular component and gliosis as a reaction to bleeding and exudation, though the main difference is said to be the lack of a specific feeder vessel and draining vessel; it just sort of grows seemingly from nothing.

Treatment is similar, though, in that, these cases are observed as much as possible and a tight watch is kept for any changes that might indicate that the macula is being threatened by leakage or retina being pulled off through gliosis. If growth is documented and there are fears for the vision, refer the patient to your vitreoretinal colleagues for cryotherapy or an ocular oncology centre if you are unsure about the diagnosis. In fact, sometimes PDT or brachytherapy is needed anyhow, so it isn't such a bad call to play it safe and refer. Textbooks will say that early retinal laser might make a difference, but we both know that neither of us are brave enough to wade in and do that.

ACUTE MACULAR NEURORETINOPATHY AND PARACENTRAL ACUTE MIDDLE MACULOPATHY

These conditions are two cousins from the same vascular compromise family. Acute macular neuroretinopathy (AMN) is the most well-known of the two and classically presents with a young female who describes the sudden onset of a paracentral scotoma. Interestingly, patients tend to insist on drawing the exact shape, as if this makes a difference to anything, and as Prof Bird from Moorfields often says, this insistence is so great that even if all pens and all paper are removed from the eye clinic the patient will take care to scratch the scotomatous shape onto the very desk in front of you. It is thought to be due to compromise of the deep retinal capillary plexus either randomly or secondary to the oral contraceptive pill, a vaccine (such as the COVID-19 vaccine), the infection the vaccine was meant to protect against (such as COVID-19), illness, caffeine or indeed anything and everything that we can think of to try to blame in bringing order to an essentially chaotic world.

There is almost always nothing to see on examination, so OCT is essential here. The outer retina is most affected and a fluffy signal is seen, usually at the level of the outer plexiform and outer nuclear layer (see Figure 10.6). These areas pleasingly line up nicely with the multiple pictures of the scotoma that the patient has insisted on giving you, and if you can ask for an infrared image of the fundus, the hitherto hidden lesion can become clear. As there is no treatment, we sometimes advise patients to give up their beloved caffeine, stop the contraceptive pill or give some other generally ineffective piece of lifestyle advice that won't make any difference to anything except convince the patient, and perhaps us, that we are doing something useful. There is no need to follow patients as there is nothing that can be done, and many patients get a little better over time anyhow. Some patients are so distressed by the scotoma, however, that you know before attempting to discharge them that they'd be horrified at the prospect and therefore some sort of follow-up is necessary, in which case, try to make it as long an interval as you can.

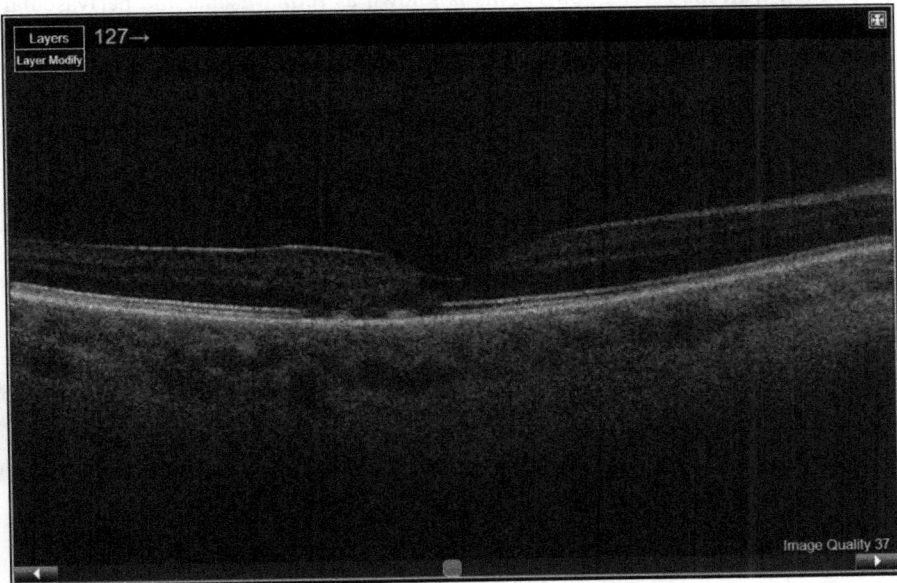

FIGURE 10.6 An OCT scan of a patient with acute macular neuroretinopathy (AMN).

Paracentral acute middle maculopathy (PAMM) is sort of the same thing but affecting the middle layer of the retina rather than the outer portion. Everything else is thought to be similar, with vascular compromise being the main cause and all the same things that are thought to cause AMN being able to cause PAMM as well. Infrared imaging similarly reveals the hidden shape that matches the scotoma, although the OCT image reveals that the hyperreflective fluffy bands are present in the middle of the retina rather than in the outer portion. Again, there is no proper treatment other than addressing any systemic conditions that might be contributing to the ischaemic compromise, but there is nothing for the eye itself.

Christiana Says...

PAMM is a retinal finding that reflects ischemia (inadequate blood supply) in the intermediate and deep retinal capillary plexus. It often presents with paracentral scotomas (small blind spots near the center of vision) and is most easily visualised using OCT. It was first described by Sarraf et al. in 2013, who used **spectral-domain OCT (SD-OCT)** to identify a **distinct hyperreflective band** at the level of the **inner nuclear layer (INL)** in patients with **acute paracentral visual field loss** (2). **It is an OCT-based diagnosis.** PAMM is thought to result from **hypoperfusion or occlusion** of the intermediate/deep retinal capillary plexus, often due to systemic microvascular compromise. PAMM is not a disease itself but a **retinal manifestation** of underlying systemic or vascular pathology such as cardiovascular and cerebrovascular disease, systemic inflammatory or autoimmune conditions such as systemic lupus, and infectious diseases such as COVID-19. In essence, PAMM is a warning sign and detection should prompt consideration of a systemic work-up, especially in patients with no known cardiovascular or hematologic disease.

In some instances, you may see focal thinning at the level of the INL, which may be aligned with the retinal veins. This is known as retinal ischaemic perivascular lesions (RIPLs), which are thought to be the atrophy left behind after acute ischemia in the deep capillary plexus. These are often incidental, asymptomatic and have similar systemic associations as PAMM (3).

WHITE DOT SYNDROMES AND UVEITIS

There are far too many to mention in this chapter to be able to cover them all properly. This would need a separate book; luckily one exists in the form of *Practical Uveitis*, second edition, by Taylor and Francis. Order your copy today!

RETINAL ARTERY OCCLUSION

As with retinal vein occlusions (see Chapter 7), retinal artery occlusions can affect either the whole retina, termed central retinal artery occlusions (CRAOs), or a specific branch, a BRAO. We tell our patients that this is a 'sort of stroke that has affected the eye' instead of the brain, and this is actually a good way of looking at this. The blood supply to the eye has been compromised by an embolus that decided to flow into the ophthalmic artery but could have just as well carried on up into the brain. For this reason, the risk factors are much the same as they would be for a patient experiencing a true stroke, or cerebrovascular accident (CVA), to use the proper terminology. These include smoking, obesity, hypertension and anything and everything else that compromises human health. Sometimes a retinal artery occlusion can occur because of spasms of the artery (rather than a true blockage), such as occurs in migraine (causing a so-called ocular migraine) or conditions such as Raynaud's disease. Lastly, blockage can occur due to vasculitis, in which inflammation of the artery thickens the wall and eventually blocks flow.

Embolic CRAO or BRAO present with painless loss of vision in all or part of the vision of one eye. Sometimes the distressed retina, which interprets everything as light, flickers and flashes, but mostly it is a patient suddenly not being able to see. As with a CVA, this is a true emergency and urgent treatment can make a difference, though sadly by the time most patients make it to the eye department, more often than not it is too late. The quicker the patient is seen the better; an hour is best, although a ludicrously unachievable target, and anything more than 24 hours is essentially too late for intervention to make a difference. Examining the patient, the main thing to note is that the affected area of retina is pale and whitish due to a lack of blood supply filling it with blood as well as swelling of the retina blocking the glow from the choroid. The fovea is thinner, of course, than the surrounding retina, and the glow of the choroid cannot be covered up, so a foveal 'cherry-red spot' is said to exist. The next thing to look for is emboli. These are of various forms, the names and description of which are essentially unimportant for your management of the patient, so just look for anything within any artery at the disc (in the case of a CRAO) or in one of the branches that could be blocking flow.

The diagnosis is obvious on examination, but should an OCT be undertaken, dramatic swelling of the retina is seen, as well as hyperreflectivity of the inner retina, which has occurred due to infarction and extreme ischaemic damage to the tissue. It's a bit like AMN and PAMM, but instead of subtle small changes, it looks more akin to a nuclear explosion in the retina, which is essentially what it is. At the time of presentation, the other consideration is a cardiovascular workup and looking after the systemic situation, so asking a nurse to undertake blood pressure and pulse measurements is wise, along with completing a referral card to the local iteration of a rapid access stroke or transient ischaemic attack (TIA) clinic, filling in request forms for carotid Dopplers or blood tests depending on your local protocol. As this varies all over the country and time is of the essence here, it is not a bad idea to make these sorts of protocols easily accessible to those working in eye casualty and to include details in any local departmental induction programme.

Anyhow, other than blood pressure and such, these things can wait; the eye is the emergency. If a patient presents within 24 hours, there is some hope that what you do makes a difference. The aim isn't to entirely reverse the situation, but rather limit the damage, to move the embolus down into a side branch to save some retina. The main thing that works here is intravenous acetazolamide 500 mg. Should this be unsuccessful, then anterior chamber paracentesis may do something, with the aim being to reduce the pressure within the eye so the arterial/intraocular pressure differential is increased sufficiently to be able to move the embolus onward. Breathing into a bag (the patient not the ophthalmologist) is sometimes done on the basis that increasing carbon dioxide levels dilates the blood vessels and allows the embolus to move, though this has more than a feel of voodoo to it. The other thing that is sometimes done is ocular massage, where a lot of pressure is applied to the eye (as much as the patient can tolerate) and then suddenly released to try to move the embolus, like a plunger in a blocked sink. This might not do anything useful, but it might be worth trying while you're waiting for acetazolamide to arrive and paradoxically, the pain this induces in the patient does give the impression that their ophthalmologist is indeed fighting for them. Nothing else is useful; thrombolysis, immediate high-dose aspirin or any other fancy intervention.

If the patient presents after 24 hours but before 48 hours, what you do is a bit more controversial as the chances of any success are slim, though you will come across case reports and anecdotes of patients being helped. On balance, it's probably best to try because the patient will feel that everything has been done, and you will feel better too. You never know, there may be an odd success once in a while, though it's best to be realistic with the patient right from the outset. If more than 48 hours have passed, then there is no justification for doing anything, unfortunately. The embolus has done its damage, the retina has been lost, and any treatment will cause more harm than good.

After the initial ocular aspect has been addressed and treatment attempted, it is important not to forget to treat the systemic aspect mentioned earlier in line with departmental protocol. It's important to bear in mind that, though rare, giant cell arteritis can be a cause of retinal arterial occasion (non-embolic, of course) and it is always important to ask about other signs and symptoms of this blinding condition. Follow-up is based on detecting neovascularisation and treating appropriately with PRP. However, compared with retinal vein occlusion, this is a lot rarer here due to the severe damage ('dead men can't call for help'), though it does occur and must be watched for at least every 3 months and for at least a year or two, though not forever.

Prognosis-wise, every so often a patient is lucky, and due to the presence of a still perfused cilioretinal artery, the fovea is saved. If the opposite is true and the cilio-retinal artery seems to be blocked but not the central retinal artery, then this is *not* typical or indeed probably in any way secondary to embolic disease. This is almost always due to ischaemic damage caused to the vasculature by ischaemic optic neuropathy, both arteritic or non-arteritic. Over time, you will observe the OCT scans becoming thinned and atrophic, though intriguingly, patients might report some kind of visual improvement, even though the vision on objective testing might be catastrophic.

Christiana Says...

In recent years, there has been a divergence in the management of CRAO in the United Kingdom and the United States, with the United States moving more towards an emergency stroke protocol approach. If presenting within four hours of the event, urgent transfer to a stroke centre is offered. After confirmation of the diagnosis, neuroimaging is performed to rule out brain haemorrhage and intravenous thrombolysis is offered. Observational studies suggest a visual benefit from this approach, and an ongoing global randomised controlled trial (RCT; Tenectaplase CRAO Study) is expected to be out in late 2025. In the United Kingdom, our approach remains early intervention with acetazolamide or anterior chamber (AC) paracentesis.

SICKLE CELL RETINOPATHY

The first written description of sickle cell disease (SCD) was in 1910 by Dr James Herrick (4). In 1949, Dr Linus Pauling published a landmark paper showing that sickle cell anemia was caused by an **abnormal hemoglobin molecule, making it the first disease to have its molecular basis identified** (5). **In 1957, Vernon Ingram identified the exact single point mutation (substitution of valine for glutamic acid at position 6** of the **beta-globin chain** of hemoglobin, Glu6Val); again, the first time a single point mutation was definitively linked to a human disease (6). **SCD** is a **genetic blood disorder** that affects the shape and function of red blood cells. It is a debilitating, multisystem disease associated with episodes of acute illness, progressive organ damage and reduced life expectancy. There are 13 genetic variants of SCD, with the HbSS genotype being most common (>70%) and most severe, followed by the HbSC genotype. SCD predominantly affects people of African and Afro-Caribbean descent, and evidence demonstrates inequalities in healthcare outcomes and access for people with SCD. Unfortunately, the early advances have not led to progress in intervention, with only two licensed treatments for SCD in the United Kingdom at present.

Proliferative sickle cell retinopathy (SCR) is the most common ophthalmic manifestation of SCD and can result in significant sight loss, although the prevalence in the United Kingdom is not currently known. Decades-old retrospective and cohort studies from other countries have estimated the prevalence of SCR in SCD patients at up to 48% and associated with significant sight loss in up to 12%.

Five stages of SCR were described by Goldberg in 1971 (see Table 10.3) (7). These are progressive, with stages 1–3 being asymptomatic, whilst vitreous haemorrhage develops in Stage 4 and retinal detachment in Stage 5 (Figure 10.7). In addition to the peripheral retina, SCD can also affect the macula (central retina). This is visualised on OCT as retinal thinning, typically starting at the temporal juxtafoveal region and very rarely causing reduction in visual acuity, although impact on other aspects of visual function are undergoing investigation. Maculopathy was not included in the Goldberg classification, as its presence only became more apparent with modern imaging techniques. Table 10.4 demonstrates the non-proliferative features of SCR.

In SCD, under low oxygen conditions, dehydration, cold temperatures, or stress, haemoglobin S molecules stick together, and the red blood cells become rigid and

TABLE 10.3
The Five Stages of Sickle Cell Retinopathy as Described by Goldberg

Stage of Proliferative Sickle Cell Retinopathy	Features
1	Arterial occlusion (vessel occlusion)
2	Arteriovenous anastomoses
3	Seafan neovascularization
4	Vitreous haemorrhage
5	Retinal detachment

TABLE 10.4

Other Features of Sickle Cell Retinopathy

Non-Proliferative Features of Sickle Cell Retinopathy

Black sunburst
Salmon patch haemorrhages
Iridescent spots
Venous tortuosity

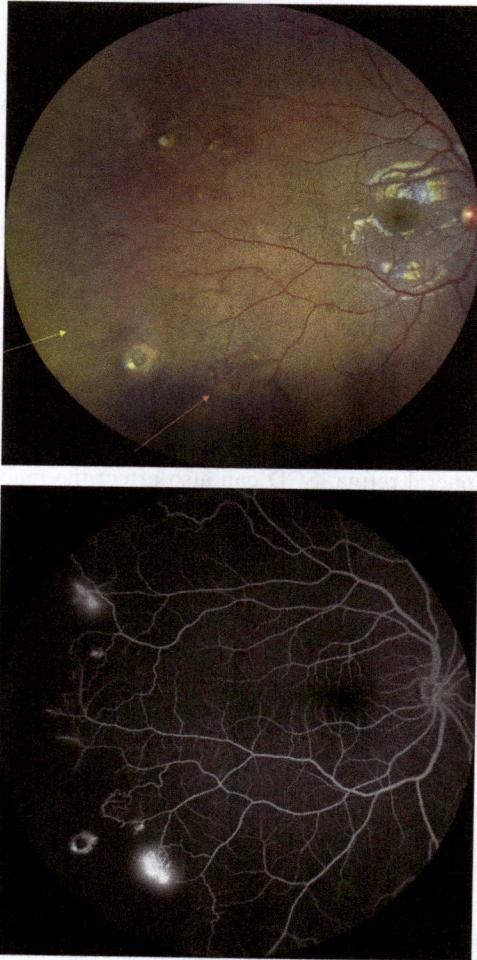

FIGURE 10.7 (a) Stage 3 Proliferative sickle cell retinopathy (SCR). The red arrow indicates seafan neovascularisation. The yellow area denotes a large area of capillary non-perfusion, which is pathognomically far peripheral. (b) Fluorescein angiography of Stage 3 proliferative SCR.

sickle-shaped instead of smooth and round. These cause hypoperfusion and reduction in oxygen delivery to the tissues. In the retina, this process results in capillary, arterial and venous occlusion. Over time, arteriovenous anastomosis develops, followed by retinal neovascularisation in some cases. This neovascularisation may bleed, resulting in vitreous haemorrhage. However, in approximately 40%, they may spontaneously regress. Some eyes progress to rhegmatogenous or tractional retinal detachment. Laser photocoagulation is currently the only intervention with high-level evidence of safety and efficacy in the management of Stage 3 SCR, the stage at which you can intervene before sight loss. Laser photocoagulation has an indirect effect because it destroys the ischemic retina responsible for production of VEGF that triggers the proliferation of new blood vessels. For SCR, unlike diabetic retinopathy, there has been a paucity of RCTs of intervention, with only three RCTs evaluating laser treatment for Stage 3, and even these were conducted over 30 years ago. These studies demonstrate significant reduction in vitreous haemorrhage and a reduction in visual loss in the laser-treated arm versus observation (8). However, the studies had significant methodological flaws, and they also demonstrated high rates of spontaneous regression. In the United Kingdom, uptake of laser treatment for SCR remains variable. To avoid vitreous haemorrhage, seafan neovascularisation that is elevated (suggesting vitreous traction) or associated with pre-retinal or vitreous haemorrhage should be considered for laser, which is applied both anterior and posterior to the lesion in a sectorial manner.

Alternatively, some clinicians in the United States and other countries manage Stages 3 and 4 with intravitreal anti-VEGF therapy. However, there is currently no RCT evaluating any anti-VEGF for this indication. Management of SCR should be in collaboration with a haematologist because systemic control of the disease has been shown to reduce the risk of progression to Stage 3 and above (9). Therefore, even if no laser treatment is warranted, the progression of occlusion in the periphery or at the macula, visualised with OCT and OCT-A, can be informative to the haematologist. The Sickle Eye Project is a National Institute for Health and Care Research (NIHR) multi-centre study designed to determine the prevalence of sight loss due to SCR in the United Kingdom, understand the impact of SCR on quality of life and influence national screening guidance for this disease. It is expected to report in late 2025.

HYDROXYCHLOROQUINE TOXICITY

During the Second World War, it was found out that antimalarial medications given to servicemen fighting in the Pacific theatre had a pleasant but unexpected side effect of helping to control symptoms of autoimmune conditions such as rheumatoid arthritis. Following this experience, hydroxychloroquine was developed as one of the main armaments used by our rheumatology colleagues, and as usage increased, a potential side effect of retinal toxicity was recognised, though it took many more decades to pass before the formal recommendation of retinal screening was advised by the Royal College of Ophthalmologists (RCOphth). The guidelines recommend that screening start after 5 years of therapy with hydroxychloroquine, unless a dose higher than 200 mg twice a day is prescribed, tamoxifen is used alongside hydroxychloroquine, there is impaired renal function, or the stronger cousin chloro-quine is used instead; in which case annual screening commences after only 1 year. At each visit, a SD-OCT is undertaken alongside widefield FAF. If both are normal, then the patient is recalled after 1 year and screening takes place again. If both are abnormal (see below), then a letter is sent to the prescriber detailing the presence of toxicity and the patient is discharged.

A quick note: The term *monitoring* seems to be favoured over *screening* when looking for potential hydroxychloroquine toxicity, and though managers and admin-istrators seem to clearly know the difference, in reality, they are two words for much the same thing, and clinicians should rightly scoff at these diplomatic and political attempts to draw some kind of half-relevant distinction.

If either the OCT or FAF is abnormal, but not both, then the patient is sent for a 10-2 Humphrey visual field test. If the field test is normal, then to be sure, a mul-tifocal electroretinogram (ERG) is performed, and if this, in turn, is also normal, then the patient is recalled after 1 year to go through the whole rigmarole again. If either of these tests is abnormal, then a letter is sent to the prescriber declaring toxicity and the patient is discharged. So, what does 'abnormal' look like regard-ing toxicity?

Classically, hydroxychloroquine toxicity caused a 'bull's eye lesion', also called a 'target lesion' because there is a normal(ish) foveal area surrounded by a circular band of pigmented change and atrophy, which, if advanced enough, would consume the foveal island as well. However, if anything is seen on clinical examination or colour fundus photography, the battle is already lost; the idea is to recognise change before such pronounced damage has taken place so further damage can be prevented. On FAF, there is a ring of hyperautofluorescence, potentially with or without another ring of hypoautofluorescence and some sort of wider peripheral change. Basically, you're looking for some sort of ring-like thing that you can't see with the naked eye. It's the same with OCT, visual field test and multifocal ERG.

OCT-wise, early toxicity is seen with ellipsoid zone disruption in an annular foveal sparing configuration around the fovea, which, when advancing, spreads to the outer nuclear layer and RPE. The classic thing is the fact that it is ring-like and only involves the parafoveal retina and not the fovea itself. There is a so-called *flying saucer sign* that is described on OCT where parafoveal disruption around an island of normality is said to cause the outer retina of the foveal area to look like an alien spacecraft from the early 20th century, but as with most of these so-called signs, they mainly cause confusion because it takes an eye of faith and some significant squinting on the part of the ophthalmologist to be able to see a flying saucer. Just look for a ring of abnormality surrounding an island of normality at the fovea. In the presence of toxicity, visual field testing reveals, you've guessed it, a circle of loss of field with a normal fovea, whilst multifocal ERG (itself a form of field test) reveals the same. It is overcomplicating things to talk about very specific findings; just look for any abnormality and see if that abnormality is ring-shaped.

Our role is to advise whether toxicity is taking place or not. For this reason, dis-charge the patient once you've told the prescriber, as there would be no purpose in following the patient and repeating the test after a year. It might even cause confusion, as the patient and prescriber might think all is well if the screening/monitoring is carrying on. It is also not for us to stop any treatment. This is the responsibility of whoever prescribed it, and eye doctors shouldn't be fiddling about with things outside their purview, for our own good.

Christiana Says...

It is worth considering the differential diagnosis for hydroxychloroquine toxicity. These include other drug toxicities, retinal dystrophies, retinal degenerations, and systemic diseases associated with retinopathy. If there is suspicion of concurrent macular disease, such as age-related macular degeneration, then the treating physician should be made aware and the risks and benefits of continuing on hydroxychloroquine discussed. It seems likely that concurrent macular disease may increase the risk of hydroxychloroquine toxicity, but this has not been definitively shown.

MACROANEURYSMS AND HYPERTENSIVE RETINOPATHY

The difference between a macroaneurysm and a microaneurysm is size, specifically the width of a vein at the disc margin. A macroaneurysm is a focal dilation in a retinal artery wider than this, which takes place within three or fewer bifurcations of the artery after it has left the disc. After this, the pressure is thought to be too low to cause an aneurysm to form. Obviously, the artery has to pass right through it as well, otherwise you will need to consider the haemangioma family (see above). Hypertension is the most common cause, so blood pressure will need to be measured and if exotically high (more than 200/100 mmHg), your friendly medical registrar on-call colleague contacted. If high but not that high, organising a visit to the general practitioner (GP) is best.

From an ophthalmic perspective, macroaneurysms have a life cycle; they form, they leak or bleed, then they thrombose, and then they disappear. Most are asymptomatic, though this depends on their location. Far from the macula is good, and close to the macula is bad. If they are close enough, then should they leak either fluid or blood, then the vision is directly involved, and only then does the patient complain. Happily, as leakage normally precedes resolution, doing a lot of nothing (masterly inaction) can be a good thing, and monitoring over 3 months can reap dividends as things start to resolve almost as soon as you've realised a leakage exists. Sometimes, however, this is not the case.

If the leakage is persistent or if acute but particularly bad, then some sort of action is needed. As with much else in the field of medical retina, if we are uncertain what to do, we inject an anti-VEGF agent, say a course of three ranibizumab injections 4-weekly, which actually seems to be associated with a good response, though this in part could be due to spontaneous resolution. Either way, the patient feels we have done them good. Some old-school consultants will talk about focal retinal laser to surround the aneurysm, and whilst this might be good in terms of pure leakage, the vision can be damaged because, by definition, such lesions will be reasonably close to the macula. If there is a haemorrhage as opposed to an exudative leak, then things are a bit different, as blood is much more toxic to vision, and so a quick referral to our vitreoretinal friends is best so they can consider tissue plasminogen activator (TPA) injection and gas or any other sort of fancy intervention.

High blood pressure is the main thing to watch for when a macroaneurysm is found, although hypertension can have many other effects on the fundus as well. Depending on how high is high, signs range from arteriorvenous 'nipping', where the retinal vein appears bulgy on either side of a crossing artery due to squeezing pressure, to a picture with cotton wool spots, exudation, and haemorrhages that looks remarkably like diabetic retinopathy or a CRVO (which might be caused by hypertension itself anyhow), to a full-blown optic disc swelling and optic neuropathy picture on top of this. Have a low threshold for checking blood pressure in such patients, though treatment is purely blood pressure reduction, which is done by the GP or medical team. Our role is to recognise it and report it to medics who can do something about it. We caution most strongly against starting any antihypertensives of our own; we are not proper doctors anymore (regardless of what you might think), and there is a risk of meddling in something beyond our ability to control and ending up causing heart failure, renal failure, or death. There might even be no point in any follow-up because whatever we find won't alter things; the only treatment is blood pressure reduction.

EVERYTHING ELSE

It would be impossible to mention everything in the entire field of Medical Retina here. The eyes are the windows to the soul, as said in the Bible, by Shakespeare, and by many others, and as such, many medical conditions have some sort of effect that is seen on fundal examination. Patients with blood disorders such as leukaemia can exhibit retinopathy, though it is the haematology team alone that can do anything to fix it. Purtscher retinopathy was originally described as being secondary to trauma, although since then, a whole myriad of other causes, such as pancreatitis and renal failure, have also been recognised as being responsible as well. The clinical picture includes cotton wool spots and haemorrhages, and treatment is fixing whatever insult caused it in the first place. Valsalva retinopathy occurs when a blood vessel bursts in the eye following a vigorous Valsalva manoeuvre such as weightlifting or trying to pass a particularly large solid stool. This is usually watched until it resolves, or we ask our vitreoretinal friends for help; yttrium aluminium garnet (YAG) posterior hyaloidotomy is usually either not possible or beyond the usual bravery levels required of a regular medical retina specialist to perform.

We have already covered the bread-and-butter conditions that we will see in clinic. There are, however, literally infinite conditions that exist. All of these can be summarised with the phrase 'do as much nothing as possible, but take lots of pictures'. This is true for much of medicine, actually, but especially here. Don't do anything if doing nothing is also a reasonable option. Don't make a name for yourself pioneering some new treatment for something if the natural history is very good anyhow. Don't do something just for the sake of doing something. Much of the time, doing nothing is fine. If you don't know what something is, just take a picture and look it up on Google after the patient has left; that's perfectly fine. If you don't know, ask a colleague. It's okay not to know, but what's not okay is to pretend to know when you don't.

REFERENCES

1. Chew EY, Gillies M, Jaffe GJ, Gaudric A, Egan C, Constable I, Clemons T, Aaberg T, Manning DC, Hohman TC, Bird A, Friedlander M; MacTel CNTF NTMT-03 Research Investigators. Cell-based ciliary neurotrophic factor therapy for macular telangiectasia type 2. NEJM Evid. 2025;4(8):EVIDoa2400481. doi: 10.1056/EVIDoa2400481. Epub 2025 Jul 22.

2. Tsui I, Sarraf D. Paracentral acute middle maculopathy and acute macular neuroretinopathy. Ophthalmic Surg Lasers Imaging Retina. 2013; 44(6 Suppl):S33–S35. doi: 10.3928/23258160-20131101-06.

3. Limoli C, Khalid H, Wagner SK, Huemer J. Retinal ischemic perivascular lesions (RIPLs) as potential biomarkers for systemic vascular diseases: A narrative review of the literature. Ophthalmol Ther. 2025; 14(6):1183–1197. doi: 10.1007/s40123-025-01148-5. Epub 2025 Apr 28.

4. Herrick JB. Peculiar elongated and sickle-shaped red blood corpuscles in a case of severe anemia. Arch Intern Med. 1910; 6(5):517–521.

5. Pauling L, Itano HA et al. Sickle cell anemia a molecular disease. Science. 1949; 110(2865):543–548. doi: 10.1126/science.110.2865.543.

6. Ingram VM, Stretton AOW. Genetic basis of the thalassaemia diseases. Nature. 1959; 184:1903–1909.

7. Goldberg MF. Classification and pathogenesis of proliferative sickle retinopathy. Am J Ophthalmol. 1971; 71(3):649–665. doi: 10.1016/0002-9394(71)90429-6.

8. Myint KT, Sahoo S, Thein AW, Moe S, Ni H. Laser therapy for retinopathy in sickle cell disease. Cochrane Database Syst Rev. 2022; 12(12):CD010790. doi: 10.1002/14651858.CD010790.pub3.

9. Smith BD, Hankins JS, Kang G, Takemoto CM, Rai P, Chen PL, King BA, Hoehn ME. Investigation of sickle cell retinopathy in pediatric and adolescent patients enrolled in a large cohort study. Ophthalmology. 2025; 132(8):911–920. doi: 10.1016/j.ophtha.2025.03.031. Epub 2025 Apr 4.

11 Service Planning

This is arguably the most important aspect of a modern medical retina service. There is, indeed, no purpose in knowing all the facts discussed in this book if your hospital has no proper means to carry out treatments effectively. We are but conductors; we need an orchestra as well, and everyone plays their part. Organising a service can be divided into what can happen outside the hospital with suitably trained optometric staff, what can happen in the hospital with the aid of qualified non-medical practitioners (NMPs), what only doctors need to do, and finally, what do only consultant ophthalmologists need to do? All this can be best summarised as 'do only what only you can do' for the best, most cost-effective use of precious resources for the benefit of our medical retina patients.

OUTSIDE THE HOSPITAL

Back in the days way before the advent of optical coherence tomography (OCT), patients attended their optometrists mainly for glasses, and extra examinations were only really concerned with obvious pathology that patients complained of or was interfering with refraction. Likewise, general practitioners (GPs) had use of one ageing ophthalmoscope with a poor battery and never dilated their patients. Each hospital had perhaps three ophthalmologists who all did pretty much every operation that was common to the specialty at the time, and the numbers of patients seen in the eye department were very low compared to today. These were not halcyon days though; instead of being seen and treated, patients were quietly going blind at home, undiagnosed, with all the suffering this brought them, their families and society.

Now we have the opposite situation; a highly educated optometry workforce dedicated to finding disease before it has claimed vision, treatments for conditions such as neovascular age-related macular degeneration (nAMD) and diabetes that never previously existed, and an increasingly educated patients who are living longer than ever and wish to retain good vision as long as possible. The only constant, perhaps, is that the poor GP still has probably the same ophthalmoscope at hand. The numbers of referrals are several orders of magnitude higher than before and with three or even thirty consultants, it would be impossible for us in the hospital to see and treat more than even a fraction of these. Regulating the inflow to a reasonable level is absolutely sacrosanct in protecting fragile hospital eyecare capacity. To paraphrase a famous saying, 'optometrists know how to refer patients to hospital, good optometrists know when to refer patients to hospital, but only the best optometrists know when *not* to refer patients to hospital'. Compared to optometry, the role of general practice and accident and emergency is now peripheral in managing almost all retinal problems.

Preventing a flood of patients who do not need to be seen from overwhelming hospital eye services (HES) can be done in three ways. First, the standard of each and every optometrist can be raised through education programmes and qualifications,

DOI: 10.1201/9781003628309-11

such as the medical retina certificate taught at Cardiff University, so they know what they are looking for and don't end up referring every patient with even a slight abnormality to hospital. Everyone has a slight abnormality if you look hard enough. Second, some sort of referral refinement scheme can be set up whereby super-qualified optometrists, such as those possessing the higher version of the medical retina certificate, can see patients with medical retina problems to assess whether they do indeed need to be referred or are best monitored in the community. Only a fraction of patients with diabetes need treatment, for example. Only a fraction of patients with some sort of macular pathology need injection. A good screening system such as Diabetic Eye Screening Wales (DESW), or local variant, can prevent needless referrals while referring those who genuinely need treatment. Third, by far the best option here, is a combination of the first two approaches.

Perhaps the only way to avoid an inundation of hospital service requests, whilst at the same time protecting patients from preventable sight loss, is to employ this combined approach. Who best to comment on this than one of the architects and teachers of further education in medical retina in Wales, Matthew Chan.

MEDICAL RETINA QUALIFIED OPTOMETRIST MATTHEW CHAN SAYS...

Modern medical retina services rely on teamwork. The most successful services don't function in isolation, they thrive on collaborative shared care, where optometrists, consultants, and other clinicians work as a unified team under strong and evidence-based clinical leadership. In these systems, collaboration isn't optional, it's essential for delivering the best patient care.

Optometrists receive excellent foundational training in theoretical knowledge and clinical examination skills. However, traditional training focuses more on detecting pathology and referring rather than management. From my experience teaching, I've seen that some optometrists can be overly cautious in clinical decision-making, not due to a lack of ability, but because they need real-world experience, guidance, and a supportive environment to build confidence.

The best way for optometrists to step up is through hands-on patient care, gradually taking on more responsibility in a setting where they feel supported, not scrutinised. Good clinical leadership is critical, not in the form of top-down authority, but as a guiding force that shares knowledge, sets clear expectations and empowers the whole team.

Yes, investing time in mentorship and training takes time and effort, but the benefits are clear. When optometrists are trained and supported properly, they can work at the top of their clinical capability, improving efficiency, reducing unnecessary hospital visits, and ultimately delivering better care to patients.

Bristol Eye Hospital exemplifies a successful shared care model in medical retina services, where consultant ophthalmologists and optometrists collaborate effectively. Optometrists receive structured training and postgraduate qualifications before practicing independently, ensuring clinical competence. Over the past 15 years, their role has expanded to include rapid reviews in anti–vascular endothelial growth factor (anti-VEGF) clinics, urgent referral assessments, and remote imaging, significantly reducing patient waiting times. Their stable presence enhances service continuity, while their involvement in consent procedures and patient communication stream-lines workflows. Innovative primary care pathways, such as enhanced virtual triaging, enable hospital teams to assess OCT scans remotely, providing rapid feedback to optometrists, reducing unnecessary referrals, and fast-tracking urgent cases like nAMD for timely treatment. This model optimises resources, improves access, and ensures high-quality patient care.

The demand for upskilling opportunities among optometrists is high, with medical retina courses being the most popular postgraduate qualifications at Cardiff University. However, while further qualifications are important, they aren't enough on their own. Confidence and expertise are built through real-world clinical exposure and collaborative decision-making, rather than solely through academic achievement. Optometrists excel when given opportunities to apply their knowledge in practical settings.

For optometrists to take on more complex work, they need structured training pathways, clearly defined responsibilities, and a system that fosters professional development. When fully integrated into medical retina services, from initial assessments to referral refinement and long-term monitoring, they can help streamline pathways, improve efficiency, and ease pressure on hospital services.

A strong team-based approach benefits not just the service but, most importantly, the patients. When consultants, optometrists, and other clinicians work in sync with trust and open communication, the whole system runs more efficiently. Supported and well-trained optometrists enable hospitals to focus on the most complex cases while ensuring patients receive timely and effective care.

As virtual clinics and emerging technologies reshape medical retina services, exciting opportunities arise to optimise patient pathways and enhance shared care. By investing in optometrists through training, structured development, and shared expertise, we ensure they are not just contributors but integral to the future of medical retina care.

NON-MEDICAL PRACTITIONERS IN THE EYE DEPARTMENT

What is an NMP? Any healthcare practitioner who isn't a doctor who sees patients in the eye department in some form of independent manner. These include hospital optometrists (who ideally are sometimes the same optometrists who also work outside the hospital seeing medical retina patients in practice), nurses and orthoptists. The role of physicians associates in eyecare is at present severely limited, hugely controversial, and won't be discussed here. To be suitably qualified to see medical retina patients in clinic in the name of a consultant, all of these NMPs need to be qualified at least as well as their community colleagues.

To use this precious resource as effectively as possible, a virtual system for seeing high-volume, low-complexity patients is useful. Because only a small proportion might need treatment, diabetic patients referred with macular oedema or pre-proliferative disease can have visual acuity, widefield photography, and OCT scans undertaken by technical staff alone. This can then be followed with trained NMPs trawling through the data to decide whether patients can be discharged back to primary care, followed up again in the virtual system, or brought in to a proper face-to-face appointment to discuss potential treatment. This is work that need not take the limited (and expensive) time of consultants, or indeed doctors of any kind. There are a whole host of other conditions that can be treated this way as well, with hydroxychloroquine screening/monitoring being another good example.

Moving slowly up the pyramid of complexity, we now come across patients who have been assessed and are deemed to perhaps need some form of treatment; let's say, a diabetic patient with vision of worse than 6/12 (0.30 LogMAR) and a macular thickness of greater than 400 microns, or some other more borderline case. Patients are best brought to a one-stop clinic from this point onwards where treatment can be delivered on the same day if this is necessary. Obviously, for these clinics to be effective and useful, only patients who stand a good chance of needing treatment are best booked into them, with other patients that need a consultation but not necessarily treatment brought to a standalone clinic without injection or laser facilities. At **both** these sorts of clinics, patients can again be seen face-to-face by an NMP.

Suitably qualified and experienced NMPs should know when patients are treated (as well as when they are not) and are able to have a proper discussion about this with them. They can also be trained to consent patients. If treatment is then needed, NMPs can carry out the injection themselves, be that intravitreal anti-VEGF or Ozurdex, and indeed have been doing this for years across the world. It is not for doctors to routinely inject patients in large volume. Doctors may have to inject for various reasons – including so that they can train others, support when more experienced NMPs are unavailable, and provide the service in their private clinics. They also need to be able to manage complications of intravitreal injections, such as performing anterior chamber paracentesis. Non-medical staff can and do inject at least as well and arguably better. The only thing junior doctors need to learn is how to inject, but this is purely from a training perspective and should not be from a service perspective. It is an immoral waste of time and money for consultant ophthalmologists to spend valuable time injecting.

NMPs may have a role in administering retinal laser therapy. This can be safe and effective and can help reduce waiting lists for laser, which is a time-dependent, sight-saving procedure. In various parts of the world, there is some protectionist pressure to restrict sight-saving procedures to specific members of staff, but do not be waylaid by this sort of pressure; make the care of the patient your first priority. What is then the proper role of the consultant ophthalmologist in this brave new world? To be the shogun sitting cross-legged in the middle of the clinic floor guiding the staff when needed, making important decisions, and arbitrating between different courses of action while training new doctors in the art of medical retina and leading the team to victory.

THE HOSPITAL-COMMUNITY SYNCYTIUM

The hospital, community, and screening system should not be siloed. In fact, they should all be one big syncytium whereby patients on their journey pass seamlessly from primary care optometrist to hospital eyecare services and then back again once stability has been achieved. Once patients are deemed stable from a hospital perspective, in that no treatment is needed from an injection or laser perspective, it is then entirely reasonable to decant these patients to primary care. A unified patient record in the form of an electronic patient record is absolutely necessary for this care to be truly continuous, but a strong primary care element makes the hospital stronger and vice versa. We are all part of the same team and to act as efficiently as possible, we all need to be on the same page concerning specific issues.

INJECTION SERVICES

Injection clinics should be as efficient as possible, following evidence-based algorithms in a rigorous and repeatable manner. These algorithms are devised by Consultant Ophthalmologists based on current evidence. NMPs are better than doctors at following algorithms. With regard to injection clinics, up to 16 patients per injector per session is more than reasonable, provided the injections take place within a suitable environment with laminar flow air exchange and proper infection control precautions. Economies of scale are key here, which is why the NHS model of hubs and spokes is so much better than the American model of office-based ophthalmology; far better to have proper facilities for injecting patients en masse with full safety precautions undertaken than doing the odd injection every so often in a far from ideal office-based environment. That said, some American-style clinics are indeed set up in a model of efficiency that the NHS can only dream of, undertaking up to 60 injections per doctor while utilising several injecting rooms and an efficient supportive team. How then should an injection be given?

Iodine. That's the most important thing. No other intervention is anywhere near as good as this at preventing blinding eye infections. If a patient is apparently allergic to iodine, then in all probability this represents a sensitivity to iodine rather than a true allergy as it affects all cells, not just microorganisms. Avoiding iodine is always a mistake and the proper and true response to patients requesting iodine be avoided is to say something like 'we will use iodine but wash it out afterward with saline'. Injecting without using iodine in this day and age, when we know its value, is simply unacceptable.

Knowing the value of something is the other side of the coin from knowing when something lacks proper value. There were several things we once took for granted in the intravitreal injection service that later turned out to be useless. The use of drapes is one. Once upon a time, injections were treated the same as cataract operations and expensive drapes were used to cover the face. Despite what you may be told by senior colleagues or infection control fascists, these drapes are entirely purposeless at preventing blinding endophthalmitis and are best dispensed with entirely. Using 10% iodine to paint the skin and 5% to instil into the conjunctival sac is the most important thing. What is the point, you may ask, of painting the skin around the eye at all? Nothing really, except that it wastes enough time so that the iodine instilled into the conjunctival sac has done its work, estimated to need approximately 120 seconds at least. In this manner, there is indeed a negative price to pay for efficiency. The only proviso is that a bladed speculum is used to keep the eyelashes away from the needle.

In the old days, chloramphenicol drops were given to the patient to use after the injection, though this has now been found to be entirely counterproductive. Don't bother. If anything, chloramphenicol makes the chances of endophthalmitis worse, though we would say it is more useless than anything else and so best dispensed with. In fact, there are many voodooistic things we do during injections in the belief that they improve things, when in fact the only thing that truly makes a difference is iodine. Iodine and efficiency.

ALGORITHMS

Whatever choice of algorithms you have in your department, make sure they are clear and easy to follow. The evidence for one algorithm over another is not as great, but consistency is key, and making sure it isn't the sort of system in which anyone can make up any sort of rule is paramount in preventing a descent into chaos. This is where the true power of the medical retinal consultant is properly expressed; it is up to us to decide upon a proper and decent way of treating things and then enforcing this view amongst the entire team. In the film *Margin Call*, Jeremy Irons plays a peripheral but important role, in which he makes decisions about the big issues but leaves the running of the company to everyone else almost all the rest of the time. 'Do you want to know why I earn the big bucks?' he says at the beginning of a crucial meeting. 'I am here for one reason and for one reason alone. I'm here to guess what the music might do a week, a month, a year from now'. This is our role. To guide the team by writing algorithms and standardising care. To keep on top of developments and make sure the department is operating at the top of its capability with the correct algorithms and the correct drugs.

Our duty is not to inject, not to review, not to provide some sort of decision-making aspect to a glorified community-based data-gathering medical retina scheme. Our duty is to lead and to lead by example. Keeping up with research and tweaking the way we do things to continuously improve practice is what a medical retina consultant does. A medical retina consultant does not make too many adjustments too often, so the team don't know whether they are coming or going, but slowly guide the medical retina ship through treacherous seas by making gentle adjustments to the tiller.

Drug choices should be based on service capacity. Longer-acting anti-VEGF agents are more expensive than off-patent shorter-acting variants, but if capacity is a real problem and appointment slippage (a real force for chaos in a treat and extend system) is a risk, then they are the only logical choice. If capacity is not an issue in your department, a very rare state of affairs in this day and age, then you could consider using the cheaper agents, though the price you pay will be more frequent injections. It becomes difficult to work out the real costs under those circumstances because each appointment also has a cost, especially an injection slot, and the patient pays their own price for attending your department more often than they otherwise might have to, especially if they are still of working age. Ozurdex injections are more expensive, but last up to 6 months (but could be as few as three), while Iluvien is eye-wateringly expensive, and though it is meant to last 3 years, sometimes it doesn't work at all. All of them carry side effects, though these are subtly different from each other.

Christiana Says...

Doctors have a role in the leadership, design and delivery of all parts of a medical retina service. If the focus is on choice of intervention, the choice of an intervention is not only based on efficacy and safety, but also on the ability for the health service in question to afford said intervention. Anti-VEGF therapies have been transformational in the West for many retinal diseases, but their uptake is patchier in low-income countries and in areas where the infrastructure for transportation and cold storage of these drugs are not well-developed. The frequency of treatment required with current anti-VEGFs requires robust administrative and failsafe procedures that can render this model of care challenging to deliver. As such, there remains an unmet need globally, including in high-income countries, for durable treatments in retina.

An illustrative scenario is proliferative diabetic retinopathy (DR), where the standard of care is panretinal photocoagulation (PRP), established in the pivotal DRS and ETDRS trials. However, this treatment sacrifices the peripheral retina to safeguard the central retina, which results in visual field restriction in some patients, can worsen diabetic macular oedema, and may potentiate epiretinal membrane. Anti-VEGF therapy has been demonstrated to be non-inferior to PRP (slightly higher letter gain versus PRP) at the primary endpoint in the Protocol S and CLARITY study (1–3). In addition, anti-VEGF therapy demonstrated less visual field loss and fewer vitrectomies. However, there is evidence of loss to follow-up with ongoing anti-VEGF therapy, with 34% lost to follow-up by year 5. In addition, anti-VEGF therapy does not modify the underlying ischaemia, resulting in progressing capillary non-perfusion once the treatment interval is significantly extended or stopped. In fact, a recent study demonstrated worse visual acuity at the return visit for eyes with proliferative disease treated with anti-VEGF monotherapy compared to PRP. National Institute for Health and Care Excellence (NICE) health economic modelling found PRP and bevacizumab the most cost-effective treatment regimen for PRP, but recommended PRP as first-line therapy due to the limitations discussed here (4). In other words, efficacy is important, but ease of translation (which is influenced by various factors) often determines whether a new treatment is incorporated into clinical services.

THE PATIENT'S PERSPECTIVE

Patients are, of course, the reason your medical retina service exists. In a famous study, patients were asked who they would like to treat them on a scale from NMPs to a world renowned expert professor, and where they would like to be treated on a scale from their own home to an international centre of excellence, with the most common response being that they'd want the top expert to see them in their own house. There is a lesson here. Doing what's best for individual patients might be different than doing what's best for all patients taken as a group. Efficient systems for seeing and treating patients are absolutely key to running a good medical retina service that delivers results for patients, but though patients may pass seamlessly through the system and their eyesight is preserved by on-time appointments with full use of virtual clinics and NMP staff, they may feel like cars on a Ford production line and paradoxically complain more than patients in an old-fashioned inefficient system when they 'see the doctor' much more often but lose sight.

It is simply not possible to have your cake and eat it too. Systems must be efficient and must make full use of virtual clinics and NMPs. It is still important, however, that we remember that although production lines save sight, people are not cars. An appointment outside the virtual clinic system, say one appointment in three with a clinician and a review by a doctor every year or so outside the injection cycle to discuss cataracts, intraocular pressure or the state of the Welsh rugby team, does have its advantages. 'How will the patient know the treatment is a success if we don't tell them?' a colleague used to like saying. The implication here is that a patient's assessment of their own eyesight is sometimes not as powerful a form of evidence as being told authoritatively by a doctor that all is well with their eyes. Make full use of the certificate of visual impairment system, the eye clinic liaison officer, and third-sector institutions such as the Royal National Institute for the Blind (RNIB) and macular society.

Christiana Says...

As we develop efficient systems, we must remember the value of research to our patients. Research is tomorrow's standard of care today, and whilst incorporating research seamlessly in pressured healthcare systems can be challenging, the benefits to patients and the healthcare system can be immeasurable. In some cases, patient participants have received sight-saving treatments when there was no other treatment, years in advance of being made widely available. In addition, treatments received during a trial are funded by the sponsor, saving the NHS millions of pounds in drug costs.

We can all take relatively simple steps to normalise research as part of our practice. For example, we can implement electronic patient records with mandatory minimum data fields for retina, which can facilitate automatic data extractions for real-world outcome studies. These systems can also facilitate undertaking feasibility for clinical trials, as it becomes easy to know whether you have the patient population to recruit to the relevant trials. Contributions to observation trials often help us understand the natural history of a disease or the efficacy of current treatments in identifying unmet needs. Whilst some clinicians will also be full-fledged academics, conceiving of the research question to generate the evidence required to inform our practice, we all have a crucial role to play in ensuring our services are designed offer our patients the opportunity to participate in research that is scientifically rigorous and relevant to their condition.

Most importantly, it is imperative that as clinicians, we can critically appraise the scientific literature to determine if it should influence our practice. All clinicians need to do the following:

1. Distinguish high-quality evidence from poor-quality evidence. (For example, is it randomized, are the potential sources of bias and confounding adequately addressed, and are the findings clinically significant in addition to statistically significant?)
2. Determine whether the evidence can inform their decision-making. (For example, is the patient population in the study similar in characteristics to the patient population in their clinic, and is the control arm the accepted standard of care?)

3. Balance the benefits and harm of any new treatment or treatment regime. (For example, understand the magnitude of the treatment effect, whether it is clinically meaningful to patients, and understand the risks and benefits and temporal nature of the treatment; in essence, view the evidence as a patient advocate.)
4. Understand the cost-effectiveness of interventions. (Thankfully, NICE does a good job here. However, cost-effectiveness can change as the cost of treatments decreases, or new data becomes available, and clinicians can be instrumental in flagging this to NICE.)

FUTURE DEVELOPMENTS

The main future development mentioned in every conference is, of course, artificial intelligence (AI). AI is meant to be the next step in medical retina, interpreting OCT scans, fundus photography, and other information to determine the best way forward. There have even been grumblings that this new technology will put many of us out of work and the rest of us to shame. For now, however, AI is still in its infancy and does not look set to replace us, although this should not be what bothers us anyway, if it is, in fact, as good as people say it will be. Our concern should be for patients, and if this development is indeed good, it is up to us to support it wholeheartedly. We should advocate for our patients before ourselves. The risk is that AI is not, in fact, as good as it is purported to be and patients come to harm; not through some Terminator franchise event where the program becomes self-aware and tries to kill them, but through mistakes and blunders that a human could have spotted a mile away.

The other big development is the evolution of longer-acting medications. Because faricimab and Aflibercept 8 mg replaced ranibizumab 0.5 mg and Aflibercept 2 mg, the search is always on for a longer-acting agent, though there are concerns after the brolucizumab-related inflammatory episodes that the more powerful agents might have some increased risk of causing serious problems. A port delivery system was developed whereby a refillable bladder of sorts was surgically implanted that could be refilled every 6 months and slowly drip feed anti-VEGF into the eye. This was a good thought, but the fact that the rate of endophthalmitis was not low was no huge surprise to anyone. For now, the drugs we have are likely to be the drugs we stay with for the foreseeable future.

Genetic therapies were thought of a few years ago as being on the verge of taking off, but this has not been the case thus far unfortunately. The technology is still being developed, but the problem seems to be far trickier than once thought. Stem cell therapies are in a very similar situation; the original cells died for a reason, and part of that was the surrounding support structure vitality. Planting a lot of trees in the Sahara won't make the desert green, but simply increases the chance of a lot of dead trees littering the sand in all directions. Implantable bioelectronic devices seem to be making some progress in allowing patients blinded by conditions such as retinitis pigmentosa to see in an extremely rudimentary way again. Whilst this is most certainly not even remotely the same as even the most awful vision in a properly sighted person, it might be better than nothing. Possibly.

Christiana Says...

Retinal imaging informs much of retinal disease diagnosis, with pattern recognition a critical skill inculcated in our residents from day 1. This makes the practice of medical retina relatively more amenable to AI than other areas of ophthalmology. AI is already playing a transformative role in DR screening, offering scalable, cost-effective and accurate methods for early detection and monitoring. These AI systems analyse retinal fundus photographs to detect signs of DR (microaneurysms, haemorrhages, exudates) using convolutional neural networks and other deep learning algorithms trained on large datasets of retinal images. These tools enable **remote and automated diagnosis**, making eye screening more accessible in **low-resource or rural areas** without specialists. Examples of systems already in use include **IDx-DR**, which is the first U.S. Food and Drug administration (FDA)-approved autonomous AI system for DR screening and **EyeArt**, which is CE-marked and FDA-cleared and used widely in DR programs. In the United Kingdom, Scotland has used a rules-based autograder (a less sophisticated form of AI) since 2011, but the diabetic eye screening programmes in the rest of the United Kingdom rely solely on human graders. There are still hurdles to clear before these AI systems see widespread uptake, and these include the need to train the algorithms to obtain high sensitivity and specificity, and to eliminate bias by drawing on diverse datasets and rigorously designed studies. Nevertheless, the potential advantages require that effort and resources are channelled to scale the challenges currently limiting widespread implementation. AI in medical retina is definitely here to stay!

REFERENCES

1. Gross JG, Glassman AR, Jampol LM, Inusah S, Aiello LP, Antoszyk AN, Baker CW, Berger BB, Bressler NM, Browning D, Elman MJ, Ferris FL 3rd, Friedman SM, Marcus DM, Melia M, Stockdale CR, Sun JK, Beck RW; Writing Committee for the Diabetic Retinopathy Clinical Research Network. Panretinal photocoagulation vs intravitreous ranibizumab for proliferative diabetic retinopathy: A randomized clinical trial. JAMA. 2015; 314(20):2137–2146. doi: 10.1001/jama.2015.15217.
2. Gross JG, Glassman AR, Liu D, Sun JK, Antoszyk AN, Baker CW, Bressler NM, Elman MJ, Ferris FL 3rd, Gardner TW, Jampol LM, Martin DF, Melia M, Stockdale CR, Beck RW; Diabetic Retinopathy Clinical Research Network. Five-year outcomes of panretinal photocoagulation vs intravitreous ranibizumab for proliferative diabetic retinopathy: A randomized clinical trial. JAMA Ophthalmol. 2018; 136(10):1138–1148.
3. Sivaprasad S, Prevost AT, Vasconcelos JC, Riddell A, Murphy C, Kelly J, Bainbridge J, Tudor-Edwards R, Hopkins D, Hykin P; CLARITY Study Group. Clinical efficacy of intravitreal aflibercept versus panretinal photocoagulation for best corrected visual acuity in patients with proliferative diabetic retinopathy at 52 weeks (CLARITY): A multicentre, single-blinded, randomised, controlled, phase 2b, non-inferiority trial. Lancet. 2017; 389(10085):2193–2203. doi: 10.1016/S0140-6736(17)31193-5.
4. Luckham K, Tebbs H, Claxton L, Burgess P, Dinah C, Lois N, Mohiuddin S. A Markov model assessing the cost-effectiveness of various anti-vascular endothelial growth factor drugs and panretinal photocoagulation for the treatment of proliferative diabetic retinopathy. Eye (Lond). 2025; 39(7):1364–1372. doi: 10.1038/s41433-025-03641-4. Epub 2025 Feb 5.

12 Morality and Ethics in Medical Retina

We are privileged in many ways to work in the field of Medical Retina. We have effective and powerful treatments in our armamentarium and can (and do) save sight more quickly and more effectively than any other branch of ophthalmology (though we are biased). Courses of laser for proliferative diabetic retinopathy, injections of anti-vascular endothelial growth factor (anti-VEGF) for neovascular age-related macular degeneration, and immunosuppressants for various uveitic conditions all save sight when in previous epochs those patients were destined to go blind. We see many patients in our service, and the vast majority benefit from our work; the cards, chocolates and various bottles of whisky or wine gifted us by grateful patients over the years are a testament to this. It is all too easy to fixate on the one or two deeply unhappy patients, for you will always have some in a busy service despite your very best efforts, but it is always important to keep in mind the significant depth of good that we do.

Why is this important? It is important because the profession is in a tailspin at the moment with services fragmented and outsourced and predatory private companies making deep and permanent inroads into bread-and-butter ophthalmic work. It is important because medical retina services are being neglected in parts of our country and patients are losing sight because of this. It is important because some clinicians do not recognise the value of their work, don't keep up with new drug developments and other service innovations, and their services and patients suffer as a consequence. It is important because we are important. All of us working in medical retina are guardians of sight for very many patients in our respective areas who otherwise would have no access to services. What we do matters, and sometimes we lose sight of this. Our role as guardians of services and systems is the most valuable of all, as we are worth many times the sum of our parts in this manner. Our patients need us.

What is the purpose of life? It is not an idle question. Why did we decide to study medicine? Or nursing? Optometry or orthoptics? To help others, we said in that interview so very, very long ago. Our moral worth as human beings is directly proportional to how we help others relative to how we help ourselves, and the mark of a good person is a positive balance on these scales of justice. There is much to be said about 'doing nothing from selfish ambition or conceit, but in humility count others more significant than ourselves. Let each of us look not to our own interests, but also the interests of others'. Are we truly free to do whatever we want in life? No, we are not, but neither should we be. As members of society, and valuable members of society at that, with the gift and ability to prevent blindness, we have a moral duty and obligation to serve the people of our communities in the best and most efficient way possible. On a personal level, we can earn much more money by restricting services

DOI: 10.1201/9781003628309-12

and opting to work in the more expensive, inefficient private sector. We can create huge demand by abandoning our public duties and choosing to serve only those who can pay, or worse, we extract money from the public purse to treat patients more expensively in a private setting instead of seeing them more sustainably and efficiently in a state-sponsored healthcare system such as the National Health Service. If we are to follow the eternal lesson 'from each according to his ability, to each according to his need' then we must put the patient before ourselves at all times. Chase not money, wealth or fame. Think of yourself at that interview all those years ago and make yourself proud.

Once we establish that we are in fact uniquely important in being able to make a massive positive difference to people's lives in this increasingly fragmented modern world, and that we have a duty to do so, then how might we best go about this? By doing only what only you can do. By leading an efficient and well-motivated multidisciplinary team of professionals based both outside and inside the hospital and by leading by example. Take joy in your work. We are very lucky as medical retina is an insanely interesting subject and we are truly blessed to be living in a time of such exciting scientific innovation. If you love your job then you will never need to work a day in your life. Medical retina is easy to love. New technologies and imaging modalities display the structure and function of living ocular tissue better than ever before. New drugs are continuously being developed that save sight. There are conferences the world over in our discipline that eagerly showcase all the newest developments and offer tantalising glints at what might be just around the corner. It behooves us all to stay up to date with these developments and to plan how we ourselves can do things differently to benefit our services and our patients.

What should we do about accepting industry sponsorship to attend conferences and events? If we are to develop services and become aware of new developments, we need to attend, and as dutiful National Health Service employees who do little private work, we have relatively little funds of our own. On the other hand, the drug industry makes many billions from selling us sight-saving drugs. So what should we do? There are strict guidelines concerning what companies can and cannot do and so long as you go into every industry-sponsored event with both eyes open, aware of inbuilt biases and subtle propaganda (outright and obvious propaganda was long ago banned), then by all means attend. The happy constant seems to be that all the big companies are equally happy to sponsor educational events at home and abroad, so spread yourself around liberally and learn all you can. Take part in research if you can; real-world evidence is particularly valuable in helping the global community of Medical retina specialists determine the best way forward. Industry can be very helpful indeed in sponsoring developments in our departments that the health boards often cannot, developments such as building clean rooms, the purchase of imaging devices, or installation of air conditioning units, all of which help our patients. So long as we are careful to avoid any prescribing bias, then we would be foolish to turn this much needed help away. It is important to be continuously on guard, however, against unconscious bias.

It is important to consider the design of our services and whether certain demographics are excluded by design, even if unintentionally. Most eye units in the United Kingdom now have electronic health records, which facilitate generation of real-world evidence to enable patient-centred service design. We have to work with our public health colleagues in advocating for increased awareness of eye health and regular optometry assessments. The evidence demonstrates late presentation of retinal diseases in lower socioeconomic groups, resulting in poorer prognosis. We also know that 'did not attend rates' are higher in people from lower socioeconomic demographics, and visual impairment is two to three times more prevalent in people from the Global South compared to those from the Global North. There are both moral and population health reasons to ensure we seek to understand these inequities and address them. This is particularly pertinent as social determinants of health are responsible for over 60% of the variations in health outcomes, with therapeutics only accounting for approximately 20%.

The majority of the novel therapeutics in retina are commercialised by industry and require randomised controlled trials to support efficacy and safety data, facilitating uptake by our health care systems. Unfortunately, many demographics are under-represented in these trials, and such under-representation can limit generalisability to the unique patients that walk through our doors. Clinical trials can be time-intensive and burdensome, which can limit participation to those with financial means. In addition, historical unethical research practices in some demographics have resulted in a lack of trust and hesitation to participate in research even when there is significant prevalence of the disease. Moreover, trials are often designed from the perspective of the researcher, with the site staff and patient participants often a second or third thought. Tests and research visits that may be surplus to requirement or could occur in primary care or at the participant's home are mandated in secondary care centres, resulting in high rates of participant dropout and poor uptake from all but the most experienced research sites. Research protocol design can also be unnecessarily stringent or vague. The medical retina community needs to work closely with industry to ensure the protocols are designed to complement current patient flows, to be as generalisable as possible whilst being rigorous and answering the research question, and patients – all patients – need to have their perspectives and priorities taken into account at every stage from research question design to implementation of the results. We need to push for head-to-head comparisons, as only then will we know if a new intervention is a step-change from our current standard of care and worth the diversion of taxpayer pounds.

We would be nothing without a service around us, without an army of non-medical practitioners working both outside and inside the hospital and all the supporting infrastructure. A general can't (and shouldn't) be driving the tanks and firing shots from the trenches. A general needs to be constantly at hand to answer questions about tactics and to make important decisions about major troop movements. As such, we, as doctors and senior clinicians, need to be approachable and friendly and at hand to answer any questions or deal with any disputes that arise. If we are off-hand with junior members of staff, get easily and visibly stressed when we are asked questions, or are rude with what we perceive as foolish interruptions, then the system falls apart. What happens then is that staff don't ask anything very much at all, make conservative decisions because they are fearful of taking unsupported risks, and the system slowly but surely starts to corrode and fail. We must always be ready and willing to help all our team members when they ask for help.

There is a hierarchy within the team as well, of course, and with enough time, more experienced members of the non-medical team can answer questions for newer ones and a reservoir of experience and expertise is built up within your service. With time, the questions you as perhaps the senior-most member of the team are asked will decrease in number, but only if we foster an open culture of asking and answering questions. Team meetings to discuss cases and service issues every so often is always an excellent way to foster a learning culture and increase everyone's interest in their work. Connecting with team members working in the community is also vitally important, as optometrists can feel isolated and alone if they do not also work in the hospital. A unified clinical record can help with this, but being able to ask questions via a secure online portal such as Consultant Connect is an important link that helps community optometrists working in medical retina to be able to ask about patients and conditions, and in so doing, prevent many needless hospital referrals from taking place. Meeting from time to time with community and hospital colleagues is vitally important so we put faces to names, and we see that each one of us is human and real, not just a name on a letter.

Senior members of the medical retina team should always lead by example. Make sure you start clinic on time, don't be late, and don't leave early. How can you expect more junior members of the team to work hard when the boss does not? Everyone gets sick from time to time, but we can all think of team members that abuse sick leave privileges and seem to be off work more often than they are in. Don't be one of those people. If, as leaders, we are seen to be always at the helm and always in work despite mild and various aches and pains that plague us all, then we should expect our team to follow suit. If, on the other hand, we are away a lot for multiple reasons, even if these reasons are valid, then we should expect discipline and hard work amongst our team to similarly suffer. Never be a hard task master, but make it clear that you expect the same respect from everyone as you give them, and work hard. We are here for our patients, and medicine is a vocation.

What about patient choice? Modern healthcare is very much pro-patient choice, but what does this mean in reality? Patients are all different. Some are very much old-school and will try their best to make the clinician decide on the best course of action, and if you ask them too obviously to make the choice, they might look incredulously at you and exclaim that 'you're the doctor!' In fact, some people will even lose faith in their clinicians if they devolve too much choice to the patient because they then erroneously believe that the clinician does not, in fact, know the best way forward. Other patients will then arrive armed with Wikipedia printouts and dubious Chinese studies about stem cells, and do their utmost to lead the conversation and plan treatment. Patients nowadays also bring their iPhones and tell us what their AI thinks their diagnosis is (particularly in Oxford). Our role is to decide what sort of patient we are dealing with and adapt accordingly. There is a sort of spectrum of acceptable choices that patients can make on certain issues, and we can guide them as much as possible but not force them to do anything. A patient with early neovascular age-related macular degeneration, for example, in an only eye who refuses treatment for nebulous reasons has to be properly understood; there is so much disinformation available online that it can take some unpacking of a patient's health beliefs to understand their decision-making process. But this is what we are here for.

Sometimes mistakes happen. Sometimes injections hit the phakic lens and cause a cataract, and sometimes patients react to our drug and their eyes become inflamed. When this happens, we have to be honest and tell them a problem has occurred and apologise. An apology isn't an admission of guilt; it is a human reaction to an adverse situation that expresses sympathy. Hiding the fact that any error has occurred at all is no good, and even worse is blaming the patient in some way by saying they 'moved', for example, during a critical part of the injection procedure. Always be honest and always be sincere.

We hope that this book has been useful to you all in understanding modern medical retina. We hope you agree that this subject is both fascinating and rewarding, with much good that we can do our patient population. As Medical Retina specialists, stewards of eyecare services, and guardians of sight in our communities, we have a very responsible and a very important role in society. We should not forget this. We have a moral and ethical duty to use our skills and our position to help the highest number of people and to put society and the need of the People before our own needs, wants and desires. We are infinitely lucky to have such a valuable role in life, and we have much to live up to. Good luck to you all and above all, enjoy what you do and keep on learning!

Index

Note: *Italic* and **bold** page numbers refer to figures and **tables**, respectively.

A

ABCA4 retinopathy, *see* Stargardt disease
Acetazolamide (Diamox), 117, 140
Acquired vitelliform lesions, 136
Acute macular neuroretinopathy (AMN), 154–156, *155*
Aflibercept, 54
Age-related eye disease (AREDS), 21, 27, 33
Age-related macular degeneration (AMD), 7–8, 36, 62
Airlie House classification, 83
Amsler chart, *29*
Angioid streaks, 72
Anti-vascular endothelial growth factor (anti-VEGF) agents, 1, 9, 64, 93, 94, 127, 140, 163
    trials, important features, **56–57**
Aqueous TAP, 18–19
Arterial occlusions, 109
Arteriovenous nipping, 103
Artificial intelligence (AI), 49, 108, 174
Astrocytoma, 149–150
Atypical CHRPE lesions, 149

B

Beckman classification system, **26**
Best corrected visual acuity (BCVA), 30, 31
Best disease, *see* Best vitelliform macular dystrophy
Best vitelliform macular dystrophy, 133, *134*
Bevacizumab, 54
Blood disorder, patients, 164
Blood glucose, 15–16
Blood pressure, 16, 102
Blood tests, 15
Branch retinal artery occlusion (BRAO), 156, 157
Branch retinal vein occlusion (BRVO), 12, 101, 103, 104, *105*, 118
Bristol Eye Hospital, 167
Bruch's membrane, 21, 72
B-scan ultrasound, 17–18, 69
'Bull's eye lesion, 162
Butterfly-shaped pigment dystrophy, *135*

C

Carbonic anhydrase inhibitors, 140
Cardiff University, 168

Cavernous retinal haemangioma, 152, *153*
Central retinal artery occlusions (CRAOs), 156–158
Central retinal vein occlusion (CRVO), 11–12, 101, 103, 105, *106*, 110, 118
Central serous chorioretinopathy (CSCR), 47, 71–72, **72**, 120–127
    diagnosis, 122–125
    management, 125–127
    on multimodal imaging, **124**
    with pigment epithelial detachment, *122*
    prognosis, 127
    treatment, important studies, **127**
Central Vein Occlusion Study (CVOS), 110
Cerebrospinal fluid (CSF) cytology, 18
Certificates of visual impairment (CVI), 32, 139
Chan, Matthew, 167–168
Chorioretinal atrophy, 64, *64*
Choroidal haemangioma, 153
Choroidal naevi, 146–148
Choroidal neovascular membranes (CNVMs), 9, 10, 37, 39, 47, 62, 64–66, 68, 70, 72, **72**, 125, 127
    secondary to angioid streaks, 72
    type 1, 38, 44
    type 2, 44, *44*
    type 3, 45, *45*
Choroidal osteoma, 69–70
Choroideremia, 132, *133*
Chronic obstructive pulmonary disease (COPD), 50
Clinically significant macular oedema, definition, **89**
Coats disease, 145–146
Coats-like retinopathy, 145–146
Combined hamartoma of the retina and RPE, 150
Computerised tomography (CT), 18
Cone–rod dystrophy, 133
Congenital hypertrophy of the retinal pigment epithelium (CHRPE), 148–149
Congenital stationary night blindness (CSNB), 133
Cosopt, 117
Cystoid macular oedema (CMO), *107, 108*, 112, 137, 139, 140, 147

D

Diabetes mellitus, 103
  type 1 and type 2, 74–76
Diabetic Eye Screening Wales (DESW), 167
Diabetic macular oedema (DMO), 1, 85, 89, 90,
    94, 99
  OCT biomarkers in, 6–7
  pivotal trials in, **91–92**
Diabetic maculopathy, 94
Diabetic retinal disease, 76–80, *77*
  tractional retinal detachment, *79*
Diabetic retinopathy (DR), 1, 11, 74–99
  diagnosis and grading, severity, 81–84, **82**
  follow-up algorithms, 98–99
  presentation, 80–81
  special circumstances, 96–98
  treatment, 84–98
Diet, 27
Disc collaterals, *109*
Disorganisation of retinal inner layers (DRIL), 7
Dome maculopathy, 64
Dorzolamide (Trusopt), 140
Doyne honeycomb retinal dystrophy, 136
DRCR.net Protocol S, 90
Drusen, 21, 22, *23*
Drusenoid pigment epithelial detachment, *27*
Dry age-related macular degeneration, 21–33
  diagnosis, 28–31
  high-risk, 27–28
  management, 31–33
  'non-exudative' or 'non-neovascular,' 21
  risk factors, 26–27

E

Early Treatment Diabetic Retinopathy Study
    (ETDRS), 3, 83, **83**, 84, 86, 89, 95
Electronegativity, 14
Electrooculogram (EOG), 14, 138
Electrophysiology, 14
Electroretinograms (ERGs), 14, 138
Enhanced-depth imaging OCT (EDI-OCT), 8,
    8, 70
Eplerenone, 125
Erythrocyte sedimentation rate (ESR), 102
Ethics, 176–180
European School of Advanced Studies
    in Ophthalmology (ESASO)
    classification, 7

F

Familial dominant drusen, 136
Fibrovascular pigment epithelial detachment,
    24, *40*
Flow cytometry, 18

Flying saucer sign, 162
Forster–Fuchs spot, 65
Fourier-domain OCT (FD-OCT), 4, *5*
Foveal avascular zone (FAZ), 10
Full blood count (FBC), 102
Fundus autofluorescence (FAF), 12–13, *13*, 71,
    122, *123*, 136, 137
Fundus fluorescein angiogram, 123
  classic choroidal neovascular membrane, *38*
  occult choroidal neovascular membrane, *37*
Fundus fluorescein angiography (FFA), 12, 30,
    37, 93, 107, 137

G

Gardner's syndrome, 149
Genetic conditions, 129–141
Genetic predisposition, 26
Geographic atrophy (GA), 22, 24, *24*, 30, 33, 130
  attributes of, **26**
  complement inhibitors, clinical trials, **34**
Gestational diabetes, 75
Glucose test, 102
Goldberg, M. F., 159
Grouped CHRPE lesions, 149

H

Hemiretinal vein occlusion (HRVO), 104
Herrick, James, 159
High blood sugar (hyperglycemia), 76
High-risk dry age-related macular degeneration,
    27–28
High-risk PDR, definition, **85**
Hospital-community syncytium, 169–170
Hospital eye services (HES), 166
Hydroxychloroquine toxicity, 161–163
Hyperlipidemia, 103
Hypertension, 27, 103
Hypertensive retinopathy, 163–164

I

Iatrogenic secondary neovascular membranes,
    70–71
Idiopathic neovascular membranes, 72–73
Idiopathic polypoidal choroidal vasculopathy
    (IPCV), *50*
Iluvien, 95
Indocyanine green angiography (ICGA), 3, 12,
    30, 137
Ingram, Vernon, 159
Inherited retinal dystrophies
  examination, 131–136
  future, 141
  and genetic conditions, 129–141
  investigations, 136–139

management, 139–141
myriad ways, conditions categories, 130
subsets, conditions, 130–131
suspect an eye condition, genetic, 129–130
Injection services, 170–171
Intraretinal collaterals, *109*
Intraretinal fluid (IRF), 120

L

Lacquer cracks, 62, *63*
Latanoprost, 117
LogMAR Chart, 88, 89
Low luminance visual acuity (LLVA), 30, 31
Lumbar puncture, 18

M

Macroaneurysms, 163–164
MacTel Type 2, features, **145**
Macular neovascular membranes (MNVMs), 46,
47, 62, 65
Macular oedema, 17, 111–113, 116–117
Macular telangiectasia (MacTel), 142–145
type 1, 142–146
type 2, 142–145, *143, 144*
Maculopathy, 74–99
diagnosis and grading, severity, 81–84, **82**
follow-up algorithms, 98–99
presentation, 80–81
special circumstances, 96–98
treatment, 84–98
Maculoschisis, 64
MACUSTAR project, 32
Magnetic resonance imaging (MRI) scanning, 18
Malattia Leventinese, 136
Maternally inherited diabetes and deafness
(MIDD), 135
Maxidex, 96
Medical retina conditions, 142–164
Medusa head CNVM, *42*
Melanomas, 146–148
Melatonin, 125
Mizuo-Nakamura phenomenon, 133
MOLES system, 146, **146**, 147
Morality, 176–180
Myopic CNVM, 65–67, 69
therapeutic agents, landmark trials, **67**
Myopic foveoschisis, 64
Myopic fundi, 62–65
Myopic neovascular membranes, 65–67

N

National Health Service (NHS), 177
National Institute for Health and Care Excellence
(NICE) guidelines, 87, 88

Neovascular age-related macular degeneration
(nAMD), 1, 36–60, 62, 65, 66, 68,
69, 94, 101, 125
classification, 37–45
diagnosis, 48–50
high-risk lesions, 47–48
injections services, 55–60
management, 50–55
nomenclature, 46–47
phase 3 trial, **59**
risk factors, 47
Neovascular glaucoma, 117
pressure issues, 117–118
Neovascularisation, 84, 111
New vessels at the angle (NVA), 110
New vessels at the disc (NVD), 77, *78*
New vessels at the iris (NVI), 77, 78, *78*
New vessels elsewhere (NVE), 77, *79*
Non-medical practitioners (NMPs), 166, 168–169
Non-proliferative diabetic retinopathy (NPDR),
84–86, **86**, 87

O

Obesity, 27
OCT angiography (OCT-A), 3, 8–10, *9*, **10**, 44,
45, 47, 66, 69, 107, 108, 125
OCT biomarkers, 59, 96
in age-related macular degeneration (AMD),
7–8
in diabetic macular oedema (DMO), 6–7
in proliferative diabetic retinopathy (PDR), 7
Ocular ischaemic syndrome (OIS), 81, 106
Ocular migraine, 157
Optical biopsy, macula, 6
Optical coherence tomography (OCT), 3–6, 22,
76
of adult vitelliform lesion, *25*
disciform macular scar, *46*
features, PCV, **51**
of macula with myopic foveoschisis, *65*
Ozurdex, 94, 95, 105, 117, 145, 146

P

Panretinal photocoagulation (PRP), 11, 15, 70,
86, 90, 93, 94, 107, 126, 145
Paracentral acute middle maculopathy (PAMM),
156
Patient-centred service design, 178
Patient-reported outcome measures (PROMs),
31, 32
Pattern dystrophy, 135
Pattern electroretinogram (PERG), 138
Pauling, Linus, 159
Peripapillary choroidal neovascular membranes
(PPCNVMs), 68–69

Photobiomodulation, 33
Photodynamic therapy (PDT), 37, 71, 125–127
Pigment epithelial detachment (PED), 24, *27*, 39, 122
Pinprick glucose test, 15
Polypoidal choroidal vascularisation (PCV), 41, 49
Polypoidal choroidal vasculopathy, 69
Practical Uveitis, 18
Proliferative diabetic retinopathy (PDR), 7, 84–86, 90, 94
Proliferative sickle cell retinopathy, 159, *160*
Pseudoxanthoma elasticum (PXE), 135
Public health, 2
Purtscher retinopathy, 164

R

Racemose haemangioma, 153
Radiation retinopathy, 147
Ranibizumab, 54, 98
Research protocol design, 178
Retinal angiomatous proliferation (RAP), 38
Retinal artery occlusion, 156–158
Retinal astrocytomas, 149–150, *150*
Retinal capillary haemangiomas, 150–151, *152*
Retinal haemangiomas, 150–154
Retinal haemorrhage, **106**
Retinal ischaemia, 111
Retinal ischaemic perivascular lesions (RIPLs), 156
Retinal pigment epithelium (RPE), 12, 21, 22, 36–38, 62, 105, 121, 123, 127, 135, 140
Retinal vein occlusion (RVO), 1, 81, 82, 101–118
    atypical causes, **104**
    causes, 101–103
    diagnosis, 104–106
    grading severity, 107–110
    management, 110–118
    pivotal trials, therapies, **114–115**
Retinitis pigmentosa (RP), 131, *131*
Retinol-binding protein 4 (RBP4), 138
Rifampicin, 125
Risk factors, 26–27
Rod–cone dystrophy, 133

S

Sarraf, D., 156
Sea fan–shaped CNVM, *43*
Secondary choroidal neovascular membrane (CNVM), 47, 49, 66, 71, 142
Service planning, 166–175
    algorithms, 171–172
    future developments, 174–175

hospital-community syncytium, 169–170
injection services, 170–171
non-medical practitioners, eye department, 168–169
outside the hospital, 166–168
patient's perspective, 172–174
Shem, Samuel, 80
Sickle cell disease (SCD), 159
Sickle cell retinopathy (SCR), 159–161, *160*
    features of, **160**
    stages of, **159**
Smoking, 26
Solitary CHRPE lesion, 148, **148**
Sorsby pseudoinflammatory fundus dystrophy, 136
Spectral-domain OCT (SD-OCT), 4
Stargardt disease, 132, *132*, 135, 138
State-sponsored healthcare system, 177
Steroids, 121
Stress, 121
Strong team-based approach, 168
Sturge–Weber syndrome (SWS), 154
Subretinal fluid (SRF), 48, 52, 120
Swept-source OCT (SS-OCT), 4

T

Team meetings, 179
Tessellated/tigroid, fundus, 63, *63*
Time-domain OCT (TD-OCT), 4, *4*
Tissue plasminogen activator (TPA), 163

U

Ultra-widefield fluorescein angiography (UWF-FFA), 11, 12, 110
Ultra-widefield fundus photography (UWF-FP), 110
Urine dipstick, 16–17
Uveitis, 156
    secondary membranes, 67–68
UWF-OCTA technology, 12

V

Valsalva retinopathy, 164
Vascular endothelial growth factor (VEGF), 22, 36, 90, 96, 104, 105
Vasoproliferative tumours, 154
Vein occlusion patients, 16
Verteporfin, 125
Visual evoked potentials (VEPs), 14
Visual field testing/tests, 14–15, 138
Vitreous TAP, 18–19
Von Hippel–Lindau (VHL) syndrome, 151

W

Welsh grading system, 82
'Wet' age-related macular degeneration, *see*
    Neovascular age-related macular
    degeneration

White dot syndromes, 156
Widefield fundus fluorescein angiography (FFA),
    11, *11*
Widefield imaging, 10–12
Wyburn–Mason syndrome, 153

For Product Safety Concerns and Information please contact our EU
representative GPSR@taylorandfrancis.com
Taylor & Francis Verlag GmbH, Kaufingerstraße 24, 80331 München, Germany

www.ingramcontent.com/pod-product-compliance
Lightning Source LLC
Chambersburg PA
CBHW052012230326
41598CB00078B/3207

9 781041 044208